The Empty Crib

My Personal Experiences of Miscarriage and Baby Loss

Charlene Robertson

◆ FriesenPress

One Printers Way
Altona, MB R0G 0B0
Canada

www.friesenpress.com

Copyright © 2022 by Charlene Robertson
First Edition — 2022

All rights reserved.

No part of this publication may be reproduced in any form, or by any means, electronic or mechanical, including photocopying, recording, or any information browsing, storage, or retrieval system, without permission in writing from FriesenPress.

ISBN
978-1-03-915587-9 (Hardcover)
978-1-03-915586-2 (Paperback)
978-1-03-915588-6 (eBook)

1. Health & Fitness, Pregnancy & Childbirth

Distributed to the trade by The Ingram Book Company

Table of Contents

Chapter 1: Why I Wrote This Book — 1

Chapter 2: Let's Make a Baby — 4

Chapter 3: My First Miscarriage — 9

Chapter 4: The Courage To Try Again — 20

Chapter 5: My Hardest Loss—Second Trimester — 34

Chapter 6: Third-Trimester Complications — 41

Chapter 7: The Impossible Choice — 51

Chapter 8: The Final Months—More Challenges — 58

Chapter 9: The Day We Finally Meet You! — 62

Chapter 10: The Hours After Birth — 69

Chapter 11: Grieving — 72

Chapter 12: The Dads — 76

Chapter 13: Closing Thoughts — 81

Chapter 14: Letters To My Unborn Children — 82

Chapter 1
Why I Wrote This Book

I WROTE THIS BOOK FOR THOSE WOMEN OUT THERE WHO FEEL alone and without answers.

There are many great books about pregnancy, and I have read a lot of them. There is excellent information in these books and this book does not replace any of them. It is not a medical resource, and I am not, in any way, a medical professional.

Every time I would talk with women about miscarriages, the recurring theme would be "why won't anyone talk about this?" and they would joke that I should write a book about what to *really* expect. Like a true girlfriend telling you there is food in your teeth and giving you an honest opinion about . . . well, anything and everything. That is what this book is meant to be and, hopefully at the end of it, you will have laughed a little and realized that you are not alone.

I believe that my story is important to everyone. It should be talked about openly and honestly with your girlfriends, your boyfriends, your mom, and your dad. *Everyone*. If it brings just one person comfort and provides some level of understanding so you feel less alone, then it will have been worth it.

Since every pregnancy is different then everybody's experience is going to be different. These are accounts of my personal experiences.

I loved the movie "*What to Expect When You Are Expecting*". It was a wonderfully entertaining perspective on the different types of pregnancy experiences, and I appreciate that they covered the taboo topic of miscarriage. I have a close friend who had the "pregnant unicorn" experience as described in the movie. It does exist, but there is a whole spectrum of experiences that rarely gets talked about. For me, pregnancy and the eventual birth experience were like a blind jump off a cliff with jagged rocks below. I was completely unprepared and shocked, never knowing what could or would happen. When I miscarried, there were no answers, and no one would talk to me about it.

This book is not meant to frighten you. If you are reading it, you may have experienced miscarriage or know someone who has. The whole experience is not for the faint of heart, but I found courage, strength, and hope that I never thought possible.

Before moving into my story, I want to say that I have two amazing children and wouldn't change a second of my struggles or pain along the way. I have strong faith that everything we go through is for a reason; however, there were times that I questioned it, cursed it, and even abandoned my faith during these experiences. If you are religious or not, this isn't meant to offend or discount. This is simply my perspective. I feel very blessed for my experiences—all my children, in heaven and the ones who stayed with me on earth. It took me over twenty years to be able to face that pain and anger.

Let's get the obvious question out of the way first: How many losses have I experienced? Twenty-eight (plus two ectopic pregnancies), of which fourteen were in second trimester and I was hospitalized for twenty-four hours or more.

I am going to be open and honest about the pain, losses, feelings, and thoughts I experienced along the way. I wrote through tears at times and often with an overwhelming sense of love. It has taken me fifteen years to be ready to tell my story. I always knew someone should write this book and I have tried for more than five years to do it—even though it has been more than twenty years since I experienced those losses and with the knowledge that I will carry that pain with me until I draw my last breath. I write this because I want people from all walks of life to be able to talk openly about their miscarriages and not be ashamed of their experiences and hopefully not feel so incredibly alone in their pain.

I will share quotes and inspiration and even the odd attempt at humour, but I want to thank everyone who has had the courage to share their stories with me. This is for all the moms out there—to all the moms who have children on earth, who have children in heaven, and who are still silently longing for children.

I am certainly not forgetting the dads, spouses, and partners out there who support these women. They have a front-row seat and feel so incredibly helpless. I openly share my husband's thoughts and feelings as he has shared them with me, including the pain he felt and how it has affected him.

Finally . . .

I dedicate this book to all my children. To my two beautiful children who have taught me so much and filled my life with such purpose and joy. And to my unborn children. They have given me such an appreciation and gratitude for what it takes to be a mom and have shown me the true meaning of a mother's love.

Chapter 2

Let's Make a Baby

AFTER A FEW MONTHS OF MARRIAGE, WE HAD DECIDED TO start our family and get pregnant . . . easy, right? For everyone else, it seemed easy—but for me . . . no freaking way!! I mean, it sounds simple. Just have sex and you get pregnant. I mean, that is what they told us in Catholic school. Stay away from the "forbidden fruit" because they scare you into thinking it can happen so quickly and easily. It is natural and every single animal in the world does it, so it is no big deal to get pregnant. That is the biggest lie out there.

For us, trying to get pregnant was months filled with exasperation and constant reminders. Social gatherings or family events became the equivalent of a proverbial punch in the gut. From the well-meaning and completely oblivious friends to the "what-is-your-name-again?" relative, the questions kept coming. "So, how come you are not pregnant yet?" or "When are you going to have kids?" or "Oh, dear, what is wrong with you?" It is heartbreaking. It seemed like everyone could blink and get pregnant but me.

After a few months, I had become completely obsessed with my ovulation and sex had become a chore. I kept trying to remember every single piece of advice and everything that I'd read. The list was endless: stay in bed with your legs up; guys wear boxers, not briefs; stay away from alcohol (seriously?); and, boom, it was a recipe for complete frustration.

After a few more months, we went to the doctor to have the awkward conversation that started with "We have been trying to get pregnant." Keep in mind these are trained professionals with years of schooling and they are considered "experts" in their field. So why the hell do they say things like *It will happen when you don't think about it?* Really, that is all we think about. Tracking this, eating that, wearing this, every second is spent worrying and thinking about the mechanics of it.

My next favourite piece of advice is: *You are too stressed, stop trying and it will happen.* Really??? Do you not think that is what the first months were about? Having midday sex and trying to have a baby is just about having sex with purpose. It is fun and spontaneous, and you have a purpose. But then one day it isn't . . . months go by, and you start to worry and think something is wrong. Then you read books and calculate your temperature and timing and more months go by . . . and still nothing.

Then you decide to ask the doctor, and this is the stupidity that they come up with. Are you new to this? Are you clueless? You want to scream at them, but you don't because you feel so completely inadequate and a failure as a woman.

They start with tests to make sure something isn't wrong with you. Sounds like a great place to start and I think that it can't be that bad. But the onslaught of tests for women is exhausting—probes and ultrasounds and so very many internal examinations.

Then you start tracking your ovulation cycles. They say this to you like you should have already known. Start charting your periods and ovulation cycles with temperatures—honestly, it looked like a bad weather chart. I had a calendar with my periods, my temperatures—both morning and night, my ovulation cycles, and the times and frequency of sex. I had a basal thermometer, I had ovulation predictor tests. I would bring these calendars and charts to each doctor and specialist appointment. It felt like I was in school again and the teacher was marking my spelling test while I stood awkwardly at the desk. He would look up at me every now and again, shaking his head, sighing, and judging me with a disapproving look. The endless questions after the studying of the charts were humiliating—Did we have sex enough? Were we doing it right? Maybe it is something you are eating? Let's try cutting out alcohol and caffeine. For my husband, too? Nope, not a necessity. I glare at him, scowling.

Then he stops coming to the appointments, so the focus becomes you. *After all, we are just trying to figure out how you are contributing to the issue*, he chides. The conversations after these appointments. Ugh. What did the doctor say? Uhm, let's see. It is my fault, and they think we are not having sex enough. Or too much. Or . . . oh, God, those conversations, and the ensuing arguments. Well, *what is wrong*? I DON'T KNOW!! Stop blaming me. You are being supportive and understanding?! Of course, you are right there every step of the way. You are awesome, honey. Sleep with one eye open tonight. Love you!

A few more months pass with more social events and the same stupid questions and pieces of advice. It seems like everyone in the world is getting pregnant or is pregnant and suddenly they are babies everywhere you look. You start to question your very worth as a potential mother. Why is it happening for teenagers, homeless people, addicts, everyone except me? What is wrong with me? Is this God's plan? I grew up Catholic, remember. Guilt is basic training. I also believe that everything happens for a reason. But for the life of me, I can't seem to figure out why this is happening to me.

Then one day the doctor says that we might as well test your husband, just to rule it out. Seriously!!! We discussed my hundred potential issues and sent me for endless tests and bloodwork and ultrasounds, the whole time treating him like a silent observer! OK, this should be good. Describe the testing for men. He must provide a sample in a cup. A sample of his seminal fluids. Well, that doesn't seem so bad. It doesn't sound invasive or painful or another two hours in a paper gown with someone's head up your nether region. I look toward my husband, who looks like you told him that you were going to tear off his head or shoot him. Why are you so freaking pale? After all my tests and things, you look pale because he wants some of your seminal fluid? Note to self: don't smother him in his sleep tonight. Wait! Is he seriously objecting to this?

Let's not pressure him, the doctor chides me. *We want to be considerate of how hard this is on him.* WHAT?? Are you even the same doctor? Am I on a twisted game show in an alternate reality? You just spent months describing how I am being emotional, hysterical, and stressed for no reason. We discussed the many ways I have contributed to this situation. We talked at length about my tilted womb and oddly configured cervical canal (still not sure what that means). We discussed how our sex positions and aftercare could be improved to increase our chances. But NO, LET'S NOT MAKE **HIM** FEEL UNCOMFORTABLE.

We book the next appointment where he brings in his sample cup, which he is allowed to collect at home. I am relieved that the spotlight is not on me at this appointment, and thankful that I won't leave it feeling so incredibly bad for once. We sit down and the doctor tells him there are no abnormalities in his sample, and that everything appears fine with his count. There isn't a need to pursue that further. So—now back to you. What? That's it? Back to me?

Let's talk about fertility options. There are pills you can take to help you become pregnant with a few side effects—increased cramping, heavier periods, weight gain, and headaches. Great, just great. Are you sure this is necessary? Will it work? I think we should try it and see if we can't get a baby in that womb—that is our priority.

Every doctor and specialist appointment just made me go home and cry. It is bad enough that you are questioning your own worth and abilities, but these appointments just leave you feeling more alone and frustrated. They would end with the same sentence: "If something doesn't happen in three months, come back." And you would silently pray that you never to have come back to this office.

Finally, one day, the at-home pregnancy test looks positive! I think it does, anyway. Perhaps I have been staring at it too long and have imagined the double line. It looks faded, but it is there—I think. I feel crazy. Honey! Go to the store and buy some more (they come in six packs at Woolco). The crazy amount of money we spent on these kits could feed a small country. *Try the pink box. Didn't we try that last time? I don't remember—JUST GO BUY ONE!!!!*

First, you must take the pregnancy test. You can't help but pee on yourself when you take these stupid tests. I remember thinking that this was a flashback to camping or when I was in college and was so drunk and trying to pee in the washroom at the Misty Moon—yep, that was humiliating. But nothing compares to the frustration of trying to see if you are peeing on this stupid little tip. Honestly, you couldn't make this bigger or include a sample cup? Oh, and when you are done peeing on the stick, you place in on the counter on a piece of toilet paper and you just peed all over it! Ugh. This is disgusting.

Now I will just stare at it and read the instructions, which are very long. It could be a double line or a partial line or WHAT?? OK. Wait two minutes. No problem—I am known for my patience. Are you sure it has only been a minute? Is that a double line or just a single line? It looks like a double line, but I will do it again tomorrow, just to be sure. I don't want to go to the doctor and be wrong again. To be accused of another hysterical pregnancy. Oh, yeah—that is the medical term for *just because you think you are pregnant.*

I thought if I could just pregnant then the hard part would be over. I would be so happy to be pregnant and it would be so wonderful . . . or so I thought.

Chapter 3

My First Miscarriage

IT IS A PERSON TO ME.

After months of dreaming and hoping and wishing, you can't believe your eyes. You stare at it. You are in shock. Is it real? Dare I believe it? It is positive. I mean there are three pregnancy tests on the counter, and they all look positive! It *is* positive!! I AM PREGNANT.

From the minute I found out I was pregnant, there was nothing else I could think about. Day and night. I wanted to talk about it non-stop. After months of trying, I was finally pregnant. I felt incredible. I was so happy. I told everyone—our families, our friends, people at work, and even random people. *Everyone*. It was a time of incredible joy followed by moments of panic. We were going to have a baby! It was all I wanted to talk about with my husband.

After the many congratulations from our friends, family, and coworkers, I quickly realized that they did not want to discuss it all the time. Although they were genuinely happy at the announcement, it wasn't constantly on their minds. But it was on my mind and my husband's.

From the moment we found out, we immediately thought of how our life would change. The thousand ways our day-to-day life would be affected by the pregnancy and the eventual arrival of our little one. It was all we talked about. We felt so incredibly happy that, after months of trying, we were pregnant—and it consumed our every thought.

After just one week, we discussed at great length what it would be like with a little one around and how it would change every part of our life. We talked about how we enjoyed sleeping in on Saturdays and lazing around on Sundays. We were pretty sure that would end after our little one arrived. We went out for drinks with work people on Fridays—that would have to stop, too.

We talked a lot about cravings and food. I wondered what cravings I would have. My mom loved strawberries and she made my dad hunt around endlessly for out-of-season strawberries. Everyone knows what their moms craved—everyone has heard the stories from their parents. I thought about everything I ate. I would ask if it was good for the baby, or if it would make me nauseous. When I was getting dressed in the morning, I would talk about how long it would be before I didn't fit into my clothes and ask my husband if I was starting to show. Hint to the partners: this is the one and only time you can safely say, "Yes, honey, I see a little bit of a bump." I mean, I know I was only four weeks along, but I was still happily checking my stomach every morning and night and every time I passed a mirror. I would unconsciously check it out and think how incredible it was that I was carrying a baby inside of me.

The other unconscious act I did was put my hand on my stomach. Constantly. When I was sleeping, standing, or sitting. All the time. And I didn't even notice I was doing it. People would comment on it and act confused. They would say that I was barely pregnant and ask why I was holding my stomach. Barely pregnant? This struck me as strange, but someone will say it—*trust me*. You are completely 100 percent pregnant, or you are not pregnant—there is no *barely* pregnant or *really* pregnant. It is simply *pregnant* or *not pregnant*. They will say it and you will smile. Other than other moms, no one will understand the instinct (yes, it is an instinct) to put your hand on your stomach. I think it is because we are protecting, acknowledging, and comforting our unborn baby. For there wasn't one second that went by that I didn't think of the baby growing inside of me.

We also discussed gender—whether we thought it would be a boy or a girl. We discussed why a little boy would be so great and why a little girl would be amazing. We would even argue when one of us would say that they would prefer a son. A son or a daughter. Our little one evolved into being referred to as our son or our daughter in just a matter of weeks.

We imagined what they would look like and what their personality might be. At this time, I started noticing my distinguishing features and those of my husband. Oh, God, not crazy about your nose. Come to think of it, your father has a giant hook nose, too. I obsessed about all the features I didn't like in each of our family members. Yes, it is true! We discussed the good and, mostly, not-so-good features and secretly wished that our baby wouldn't have Uncle Fred's giant ears or his dad's hook nose. Then I would start to panic about what our child could look like, and would describe a baby with all these undesirable features to my husband. I would stare at him with such panic at the idea of it and he would laugh. It caused a few heated arguments and inspired some lively discussions that would last for hours. But we couldn't stop talking about it. Our baby had these imaginary features, and we were picturing in detail what they could look like.

It had only been a few weeks since the positive pregnancy test, and we were even discussing the baby's personality traits and what they might be like. We discussed—in depth—our family members' personality traits. If you think the physical characteristics discussion was a fun and frightening one, the "wonder what they will be like and who they will take after" was an even more intense conversation. What do you mean you don't want them to be like my brother? We started picking apart each of our family members and no one was excluded. This also led to long and lively debates and conversations. We were imagining and arguing about the personality of our baby. This is important because they had once again evolved in our minds. We had imagined what they would look like and now we were discussing their personality. They had become a very real person to us.

It seemed only natural that our discussion of our baby included what type of parents we wanted to be. *I am not going to do this like my mother, or your mother.* And the lively discussions started again. We were picking apart everything and imagining every possible scenario. This was a time of great personal insight and growth because I started to really look at myself as a parent. I started to think of myself as a role model for this baby and now I was something more than the person I had been the month before.

We started to picture what our days would look like with our child. We would imagine taking them to the neighbourhood park we had driven past a hundred times without looking at—until now. We talked about swimming lessons and the type of activities in our neighbourhood. When we went to the gym, I started to investigate whether they offered children's programs. We would visit pools and facilities with children's programs. We imagined doing everything with our child and our view of the world was changing. We were viewing everything in relation to our child. We were noticing crosswalks in our neighbourhood and children playing in the neighbours' yards. Our world had expanded in a very short time, and we looked at everything differently.

We even started to discuss schools and family vacations. There wasn't a part of our life that we hadn't thought about and we knew everything would be different from this point on. It was both scary and exciting to think about. It hadn't even been a month since we found out and we had integrated this person into every part of our daily lives and neighbourhood. We couldn't believe that, in such a short time, we had discussed what they would look like, what they would be like, and what we would do with them. We had turned up every corner of our life and made room for them. We had completely changed how we looked at every aspect of our lives and discussed and imagined this in grave detail. All before we were even eight weeks pregnant. This baby was already a part of our every waking moment and every thought. It was the first thing I thought about in the morning and talked about with my husband and the very last thing on my mind every night before I fell asleep. It was an all-consuming feeling of elation and excitement that was unequalled to anything we had experienced before. I soon realized that my every thought had one common theme: *Is this good for my baby?*

My baby!

Waves of excitement filled me when I thought of my baby. My hand would immediately go to my stomach, and I would have this giant smile on my face.

This one thought consumed me, and it was incredible. This was complete joy and happiness. It filled me with such purpose and such completeness. I was more than just a person; I was a mom. There was an actual person growing inside of me and this fueled my every nerve, emotion, and thought.

I was obsessed with finding out everything about pregnancy and this life growing inside of me. I loved to read, and I wanted to read every possible book that had ever been written. I went to the library and checked out everything. I wanted to know *everything*. Every night, I would sit and read from my books and announce my findings to my husband. *Did you know we are growing organs this week? The heart is fully developed—wow! It has a heart, and it is developed!* The development of a baby is quick and amazing. We were completely consumed with the thought of our baby.

One of the things I immediately noticed when I found out I was pregnant was that smells were heightened. This is not a convenient time for this to happen, as the smell of everything made me nauseous. I could smell a KFC from a mile away and, thirty years later, that smell still makes me nauseous. I worked in a mall and the many smells coming from that food court were an onslaught. I could smell the grease in our third-floor offices. Someone would walk in the office with a burger or a donair and I could smell it instantly. It was so powerful that I would have to run to the washroom. There were times when this nausea was constant and so powerful that all I could do was eat saltines and drink ginger ale. Anything else would send me immediately to the washroom. I hated throwing up and I did it constantly for the first few months. They call it *morning* sickness and I am not sure why. It was every time of the day—morning, afternoon, evening, and even in the middle of the night. Nothing I read in my pregnancy books about morning sickness came close to describing what I felt every second of the day.

As overwhelming as the nausea was, the exhaustion was just as bad. It said in my pregnancy books that you *may* experience *some* tiredness. Scratch that out and write, "You *will* experience *complete and utter exhaustion all the time.*" It was like I had become narcoleptic. Keeping my eyes open during the day became impossible. The exhaustion that immediately overtook my body was incomparable. I literally wanted to sleep all day. It was overwhelming. It seemed like my nausea made me exhausted, but I couldn't sleep because I was always nauseous. It was an endless loop.

I know I make it sound awful, but it really wasn't. The weird part was that I was filled with such joy and excitement about the baby that I didn't mind. The constant tiredness and nausea were tangible proof that I was pregnant and that there was life growing inside of me. I know this sounds completely insane and, honestly, a complete mystery. But the moms are all laughing and nodding and saying "yes, it is true." I think from the moment I found out I was pregnant; I became a mom. My every thought revolved around my baby, and I was completely obsessed with the baby's health, emotions, and everything.

And then it happened ...

With no warning or any indication, I went to the washroom for the twentieth time that day and it happened. There it was. Blood on the toilet paper. It was unmistakable and in an instant panic and fear set in. There wasn't supposed to be bleeding. Some spotting is normal in the first trimester, but not bleeding. And this was definitely bleeding. I could not catch my breath. The world had stopped. I lay down and started to wish it away or pretend it didn't happen because it was completely overwhelming. Then as I was lying there so still and unsure if I was breathing, I noticed a cramp. Oh, God! Was that a cramp or a pain in my lower abdomen? It couldn't be!

Time passed, maybe an hour, and I was still lying there. Maybe I should go to the washroom again. But I didn't want to because I didn't want to see the blood again. Maybe it was a one-time thing, and I was imagining this cramp in my stomach. I could not let it even enter my mind, what could be happening. I could not let myself think about it. I frantically reached over to the nightstand and started to flip through my books. Yes, here it was—some spotting is normal in the first trimester. Was this spotting? It could be spotting. If I went and checked and the bleeding had stopped, then it was just spotting. Nothing more. I slowly got up and just kept repeating that everything was OK. I went to the washroom again and wiped. Took a deep breath and looked. Oh, no!! I was still bleeding.

I called my husband—*I think something is happening. I am bleeding. I know it isn't normal. I don't know why it is happening. I didn't do anything. I don't know what to do. I feel so helpless and all I can do is just sit on the floor and cry. Why does everyone assume I have this automatic download of information?*

Meanwhile, the cramping was getting worse. This felt like a rock in my stomach. What was going on? I went to the washroom and checked. I was still bleeding!! In my mind, I started to go through everything I ate that day. Nope, nothing out of the ordinary. Then I reviewed everything I'd done in the previous twenty-four hours. Maybe because I took the stairs yesterday instead of the elevator? Could that have caused it? I was feeling tired yesterday and I should have gone home. Was this it? Should I have stayed at home and rested? Would that have made a difference? As I sat on the bathroom floor with my hand on my stomach, I continued to berate myself and begged and pleaded that everything would be OK.

Had I caused this?

Was this because, when I was throwing up yesterday, I said I wished it would stop? I meant the throwing up. I didn't mean anything else. Oh, God. I am so sorry! I didn't mean it. I would throw up a thousand more times if this wasn't happening. I was now crunched on the bathroom floor because the cramps had become so bad. This was so painful, and I just wanted it to stop. I was grasping my stomach and lying on a towel because of the bleeding. The pressure in my stomach was worse than any flu or period cramp. It felt like someone was pushing on my stomach. Was this a miscarriage? I'd heard about those but had never given them a single second of thought.

This cannot be happening. I cannot be losing my baby.

We had plans—we were looking at cute baby outfits just last week. For our baby. For my baby. I promised I would look out for them—I promised it was going to be great. I told the little one I loved them and couldn't wait to meet them.

My husband was banging on the bathroom door. *No—don't come in. You can't do anything. Call the doctor. Call the hospital. What do we do? What can I do to make this stop? This pain is so strong, and the cramping is really bad now. The pressure in my stomach is so intense.* Suddenly, it felt like my insides fell out and not just all at once. It kept coming. The clots kept coming out of me! No. Stop! Don't leave! I stared helplessly at this giant blood clot on the towel. No—it couldn't be. The bleeding continued and there were more clots. I was screaming and not because of the pain because I was losing my baby and I couldn't do anything to stop it. I was oblivious of my husband screaming at the door.

Then it stopped. The bleeding and the pain stopped. I just lay there, unable to move, staring at the clots on the towel. *Oh, God, what do I do?* I called to my husband, who had been on the phone with the hospital, desperately trying to get some answers. They said to come to the hospital if the bleeding or pain got worse. *Honey? Is the bleeding worse? No, it has stopped, I say, weakly.*

I wasn't leaving that bathroom. *Oh, God, I think I lost our child. How can this have happened? Let me in*, he says. *No—you don't want to see this. Please,* he says, *I can't just stay out here.* I opened the door. He was shocked by the blood on me and then he saw the clots on the towel. I was collapsed on the floor, crying.

I lost the baby. *Oh, God. I lost our baby.* He asked me *how. What happened?*

I don't know. I don't know. I couldn't stop it—I tried, but I couldn't.

What did you do?

I don't know. It just happened. I have no answers. The books didn't say anything about this.

He ran the tub and suggested I wash up. *No! Don't touch me. Don't touch the baby. What were you going to do? Just flush it down the toilet. like a goldfish? You can't. It is our baby.* I started to rant. *I am sorry—I really didn't care if he had your nose. It isn't that bad. I am sorry I said anything at all.* Did I lose the baby because I was ungrateful or worried about silly things like looks? I was not being silly—what was I supposed to think? How was I supposed to make sense of this? Our baby was gone. I was yelling at him that he didn't care and that he didn't want to talk about it as much as me (which I knew wasn't true). But I was mad, and I felt so helpless. I cried as I washed the blood off my legs in the tub. I was beyond sad—I felt empty. I had lost my baby. *Kittens have babies. Everybody has babies, and I couldn't do that right. How could this happen? What did I do wrong? Why did this happen to me?* I felt so alone and ashamed. I just sat and cried. I put my hand to my stomach and the baby was not there anymore. It was gone. I had lost it. I crawled into bed and was so numb.

I was still tired and sad when I woke up the next morning. Just this overwhelming, deafening sadness that neither one of us could talk about. We just looked at each other. Suddenly, the weeks of conversations about the little one—the non-stop excited chatter—were replaced by an empty silence. I looked at the stack of books. *Put those away and take them back to the library! I don't want to see them again. How can I forget that this happened? How can we come home and not talk about this for every second?*

I went to work because I wasn't sick and sitting at home alone in my sadness and emptiness would be too much. It would swallow me whole. I felt like an empty shell. It was so hard to face everyone. It was embarrassing and I felt shame. I had no answers and no explanations. I had never experienced this before, but I wasn't prepared for what everyone said. I expected them to console me, comfort me, and tell me how sorry they were. But they said things like "At least it happened now" and "guess it wasn't meant to be." *How could they say that?* Well, it was only the size of a peanut—nothing to miss there. I stared blankly at people for their incredibly insensitive and stupid comments. But they were blissfully and completely unaware of how much this baby had affected over lives over the previous few weeks.

We changed everything—even ourselves. We wanted to change everything about our lives and now there was just emptiness. It may have been the size of a peanut, but it had a fully functioning heart that stopped. It had a heart and organs and then it was just a giant clot on my bathroom floor. It wasn't nothing—it wasn't just a peanut. It was my baby—*our baby*. I was a mom—I was going to be a mom. But no one wanted to talk about it. No one wanted to acknowledge our loss. No one even seemed to acknowledge that we had even lost anything. How could they possibly know that we had lost *everything* the night before? We had vacations planned and family activities. We had been talking about walking in the park and having Sunday afternoon picnics.

Now I had to smile like it didn't matter. But it *did* matter. It mattered a huge deal to us. We had talked about names. This was very real to us. *This was a person.* We were grieving the loss of our baby and it didn't matter how big it was and that no one even thought it was a baby.

I wondered if my husband was getting any more support. He wasn't. When he told them that we had miscarriage, it was a passing remark to them with a few more insensitive comments and jokes. It was clear that we were alone in our grief. It didn't matter if no one thought it was a baby. *It was to us.* I wanted to talk about it. Every time I brought it up, people would say it was better this way. *They are with God now.* I couldn't accept it. I wanted to scream at them. It was not better now. This was terrible. God didn't want this—He wouldn't take my baby away from me and put me through this. This wasn't the God I knew. He was loving and wonderful and He doesn't just steal your baby away. Rip it from you without any reason. That night, I said to my husband, "It feels like this wasn't real for anyone else. That it was no big deal we lost our baby."

I had to acknowledge the baby—I had to let them know I missed them. We had to mourn them. Even if it was just privately. *I think it was a boy*, I said. *Me, too*, he said. *When I was going through baby names, I saw Matthew and it means gift from God. Can we call him Matthew? A gift from God, so we know he is with Him in heaven now and happy? That is a great idea. I think he would have had blonde hair and blue eyes, don't you? Absolutely*, he said. *Do you think he knows we wanted him so much? That we would have loved him so much? I want to write him a letter so that he knows that. Does that sound OK? Yes—we can bury the letter with the baby clothes we bought. How does that sound? We lost our baby and I feel like we need to say goodbye.* On that sad evening, we both said our final goodbyes to Matthew, who would always be in our hearts and minds. I thought about meeting him one day in heaven. It made me smile.

When we met with the doctor, we expected him to be shocked or upset. He would know and understand what we went through. He would give us some answers as to why this had happened. Instead, he just said that *these things happen*. About 20 percent of pregnancies end in miscarriages. Quoting statistics always makes people feel better. *Just wait a few months and try again. Everything looks fine, so it looks like you expelled everything.*

We walked out of the doctor's office in silence. We drove home in silence. We sat down on the couch. I was so stunned. Then I started to rant. "Expelled everything," like it was a bad poop or something bad I ate? Just try again—just hop on that bike and try again? Like it was *that* easy—like it was as simple as doing it again. *But it wasn't that easy. It was our baby.* For the next two months, we mourned and sat in quiet over our loss that the world didn't acknowledge or see. Even his family acted like it was a set of lost keys—or of less importance. *These things happen* became a familiar response. We felt as though we had these big gaping holes in our hearts where our baby had lived—and no one even saw them.

Eventually, we stopped talking about it. But I never stopped thinking about it. It was just as hard for my husband to talk about. *We can try again*, he said. *Sure*, I said. No big deal—except how do you do that? How could I be brave enough to try again? To get pregnant again knowing that miscarriage was a real possibility now. We thought we had known what could happen. You get pregnant and have a baby—simple, right? It was different now. Now I knew you could get pregnant and not have a baby. That you could lose that baby and it would seem like the whole world didn't even notice. You just move on and try again.

Only . . .

It was a person to me.

Chapter 4

The Courage To Try Again

EVERYTHING CHANGES AFTER A LOSS.

Pregnancy wasn't the end of our worries; it was just the beginning. I hadn't even thought that miscarriage was a possibility before, but now I knew what could happen. *You get pregnant and have a baby* is the public mantra. But it was like we knew this terrible secret. You can get pregnant and *not* have a baby. I had heard of people having miscarriages, but this was unlike anything I could have imagined. We knew how hard it was to experience such loss and we had no answers as to why it had happened.

How could we even think about becoming pregnant again? To knowingly face that risk again. We were terrified. It was a fresh wound and even though we couldn't voice it, all that pain was still there. My husband didn't want to go through that again and he didn't understand why I would think about putting myself through that again. But no matter how hard I tried not to think about it, the simple fact remained that I still really wanted a baby. I convinced myself that we wouldn't have another miscarriage. One miscarriage happened, but two miscarriages seemed extremely unlikely. The doctor encouraged us to try again. *These things happen and there was no reason to believe it will happen again*, he told us. I had convinced myself that this was true and had persuaded my husband to try again.

When I finally became pregnant again, it was a mixed bag of feelings. There was joy and fear. The first time was just joy and the blissful outlook of "We are having a baby." The second time, I tried to remain optimistic and happy for my husband and gave him my best cheerleader speech of how great everything was going to be.

My feelings and fears about being pregnant weren't the only thing that had changed. My husband didn't want to talk about it as much as the first time. The nightly conversations were short or non-existent. He was scared and didn't want to think about it, so he didn't want to talk about it either. We weren't celebrating milestones and the development at every week. It was different for me too. It wasn't like the first time. Instead of reading to find out about this amazing life growing inside me, I became obsessed with finding out what could possibly harm the fetus. I kept these feelings to myself and started to feel alone in the pregnancy.

He was also cautious and hesitated to tell people this time. It wasn't like the first time we got pregnant and told everyone we were going to have a baby. We miscarried. He wanted to be sure and wait until we were three months along. I wasn't prepared for that reaction. The first time, you call everyone and share your great news and, this time, you hid it. When we did tell everyone, they echoed caution, reminding us of what had happened. The most shocking thing for us was how things had changed for everyone after our first miscarriage. People had dismissed it afterward with apathy and passing comments about trying again. What we were not prepared for was everyone's reactions when we *did* become pregnant again. They didn't want to talk about it or acknowledge it. My feelings of loneliness grew, and I felt like I couldn't talk with anyone.

It is different going to see the doctor after you have had a loss. The visit isn't full of excitement and positivity. There is concern and caution and the tone of your appointments is different. It was surprising to me as the doctor had encouraged us to try again and had stated emphatically that miscarriage was more common than we realized. At the first appointment, though, he listed the many things we should do to ensure a healthy pregnancy. He asked questions about my history and inquired about my feelings toward the pregnancy. It felt more like a cross-examination than a pregnancy appointment. I began to dread these appointments. Instead of viewing them as important milestones in our journey, they were something to endure. They offered no consolation or words of encouragement and no answers. I always left feeling more worried and defeated.

And it did happen again. We miscarried.

We stopped discussing that we were trying to have a baby after a few miscarriages. It became too hard to have those conversations. It went from "let's have a baby" to "let's try again" to "are we really going to go through another miscarriage?" Having a baby seemed like an impossible dream.

After about a dozen miscarriages, taking the pregnancy test is a different experience. I remember taking the pregnancy test and holding my breath. I was so afraid to even look at it. I finally mustered the courage and, suddenly, was frozen on the floor—afraid to move. This paralyzing fear overcame me. There was this precious cargo inside me. There was a baby inside of me. I couldn't move. I had to be so careful this time. I carefully stood up while death-gripping the positive pregnancy test. I made it—I was standing! My hand instantly went to my stomach. Are you OK, little one? What? Had I just said it? *Little one?* There was a little one inside of me. Yes! *You are going to be alright; I promise. I will do everything I can to protect you. I will do everything right and I will make sure you are born. I will get to meet you and see your face.* I started to cry again—*please, God, don't let me break this promise to this little one. I can't go through another loss—I am not strong enough.*

Oh, no! I had to go to the washroom—I had to pee. *OK—breathe. You pee lots. Don't check the toilet paper for blood. It won't happen this time. Push it out of your head right now!* I was trying to be so brave, but the fear was there. I checked. No blood!! Hooray! We made it—*you are still OK.*

Be happy—enjoy this moment! Think of the little one. You want to be able to tell them how happy you were when you found out. Remember this moment right now—on the bathroom floor, holding the positive pregnancy test. Remember how happy and full of joy you felt—you will tell them about that. You cannot think of what could happen—you can't dare think of it and can't tell them you thought of it. Right now, just enjoy that this little one is here. You can't think of the losses—you don't ever want to tell your baby that you didn't think they would make it. I had to 100 percent think that this pregnancy was going to be a baby. I couldn't allow myself to believe otherwise. I couldn't allow that thought to even enter my mind. Nope—*I 110 percent know you are going to be born, little one! This time, I know it—I can feel it. I know I will get the chance to meet you.* This is what I will tell them when I meet them for the first time. When I saw their little face and looked into their eyes, they would know I believed this would happen.

Even if it seemed like the whole world didn't think they would be born, I had to believe it. I needed to believe it. *I will believe in you, little one—I will protect you. I believe—I really believe.* I started to cry as the joy and relief set in. I was so happy, and my heart felt so open. I would allow my heart to open to the deep love I felt for this little one. I would always remember this moment—the first time I knew they were there. I would tell them all about it. *I remember the very moment when I found out I was pregnant with you, little one. I was so happy—I was so filled with joy. I cried. I loved you from that moment and I believed.*

I could not think about the past. I could not think about the previous ones. I just had to think about this beautiful miracle and how much I would do anything to protect them. How I would give anything for them to be safe and happy. This is what it feels like to have a piece of your heart truly a part of someone else. The intense joy and instant connection you feel—like your heart suddenly splits in two and you freely gave it away. It is the scariest and most wonderful feeling in the whole world. I believe this is a connection that only a mother can feel. I am not saying that the dads don't hurt or feel joy for this little one. They *do*—immensely and deeply. But this little one is in *your* body. You have been trusted with this life—to protect it, to keep it healthy. *We*—yes, we—are a team now. The little one and me. We just need to make it through thirty-six more weeks.

OK—let's just think about the first three months—what did that doctor say? All the development happens in the first three months and if you make it past then, their chance of survival goes up. So, let's just concentrate on getting through the next eight weeks. That feels overwhelming and scary. All right, let's think about getting through the next four weeks—the next week—the next day. Day by day. That sounds right.

I tried to shake off the panic and fear of what could happen thinking of the little one inside me—I would be brave for them.

Panic started to creep in. I had to go to the doctor to confirm it. *Not the doctor again. Last time he gave you that look and that head tilt. He will caution you about getting your hopes up, given your history.* My history. He means my miscarriages. After a few losses, you are considered a 'high-risk' pregnancy and just about everything changes from a medical perspective. There is a feeling of shame after each miscarriage and a feeling of impending failure to announce another pregnancy. The doctor subtly questions if there are things that you are doing to affect the pregnancy outcome. So, you stop sharing any fears and stop asking questions.

How do I tell my husband? He was so upset last time. Will he be excited? Will he allow himself to be excited or will he look at me, preparing for the worst again? Panic. Fear. Excitement. Hope. It was all there. I wanted to scream it from the rooftops, but I wanted to keep it a secret. A well-guarded secret from the friends and family—oh, the well-meaning family. *This isn't fair, you think to yourselves.* When women get pregnant in the movies, it is a time of joy and celebration and not one single person gives you that pathetic look of sympathy. *Let's focus on the positive—nope, you can literally feel all the doubts and judgement. The comments like "We will just how this one goes" leave you stunned. Did you just say that? We will see how it goes. I am sorry, was that tough on you? You refuse to believe I am pregnant because it was so utterly devasting for you? Nope, pretty sure it was just glib comments of "oh, well," it has happened to you before. Not a surprise, really, and they go on with their lives. No big deal. But it was a big deal! We cried for weeks—every time I thought about my baby—yes it was my baby—it was this stabbing pain in my heart. But no biggie for everyone else—acting so glib and nonchalant.* The responses and comments from friends and family only added to the hurt.

He is home. Just tell him. You can't keep him from this. You know that he is one person that will be as happy as you are. This is the only person you can share this with who will be happy. I need him to be happy and to believe. That is my strength, and I can get through this if he is happy and believes. Hey, honey—guess what? You show him the positive pregnancy test. He looks at it. Are we? Yes, we are! A blank stare—NO! You are happy right hon? Of course. Let's be cautious. We just can't get our hopes up again. What? No. You are supposed to believe and be happy. You can't think like that. This is a happy time. Why aren't you sweeping me up in your arms and telling me how happy you are? Why aren't you talking to my stomach and telling the little one that you are happy? You just walk away and make supper.

I was sitting there feeling so alone. But I was not alone—I had the little one now. I would be brave, and I would be strong. *If your father doesn't believe just yet, I will believe for the both of us. Don't cry. He is just being cautious. This is supposed to be a happy day in our marriage. Months and months of trying and you can't give yourself this one freaking day to rejoice and dance around. It is not fair. It is just not fair.*

What? Did you say something? Oh—you don't want to tell anyone—not for another couple of months? Let's just see how it goes. Makes sense. Why does this feel so sad—can't we just be happy for tonight? Can't we just let ourselves believe? My husband tells me to just put it out of your mind—don't think about it. "It works for me. I just stop thinking about it," he declares. Then it strikes me—that is the difference between a mother and a father. A mother is a mother from the moment she finds out she is pregnant. The baby inside of you is real and consumes your every thought. Really, you can do that. You can stop thinking about this little one completely? I can't—not for a second, as I realize my hand is still on my stomach. I don't want to stop thinking about the baby.

I can't stop thinking about you—I won't stop thinking about you. Don't worry—we are in this together. I will never leave you and I will never stop thinking about you. That night when I fall asleep, I will remember this day as the most wonderful day! This is the day I found out I was going to be a mom. Good night, little one—I love you.

The next morning when I awoke, my very first thought was of the little one. *Good morning! How was your night?* You feel like you have this big, amazing secret and you are bursting full of happiness.

"Hey, honey—how are you feeling? Can you believe it?"

"What do you mean *what*? You forgot? We are pregnant!!"

"I told you I am not thinking about it," he snaps.

It feels like a punch in your heart. *Really? Don't let him see you cry. Just go to the bathroom. We are pregnant. We are pregnant. No, WE are not! I am. I am pregnant. Because I can't stop thinking about it—I don't want to. I want to think of my little one for every second of everyday.* I worry about them everything time I go to the bathroom—I check each time I wipe for the slightest hint of blood on the paper. Every second of every day. I think to myself: is this good for the baby? Is this really what it is like being a mom? This constant worry?

No coffee this morning. Caffeine can cause miscarriages, so, nope. Ugh, this day is going to be rough to get through. No Advil or Tylenol for the inevitable caffeine headache because it could cause miscarriage. Let's review how our life changes from this day forward. No strenuous activities, so stop going to the gym. No walking up stairs—we just take things easy. No straining going to the bathroom. Nothing that would even—could even—cause anything to happen. Tell me again to just put it out of my mind and not think about it. I can't, because I need to think of how everything I eat and drink and do affects the pregnancy. It is simply not possible. It is different for husbands—they can still have coffee and Advil and not think about your every little move or thought. Just breathe—don't panic. Don't want to stress the baby—extra stress on Mother means extra stress on baby. OK—breathing again and crying! I feel so alone. I can't tell anyone. I can't talk to anyone, not even my husband. We are pretending it doesn't exist.

Every pain in my stomach—sheer panic—did that mean something? Was that a cramp? Oh, God, no! What was I doing? Nothing—no, everything is OK. It isn't a cramp—it is just gas. Seriously, I had a panic attack over a fart! But, hey, let's not think about it. How was your day? Fine—great. I think I will go to bed and rest. I am tired. I know we are not thinking about it or talking about it, so I will just pretend I had a long day. I won't tell you about my caffeine headache or my general feeling of tiredness. I am mentally exhausted, and it has only been one day. But we made it. It is OK, little one. It will be OK—we made it through today and we will make it through tomorrow and all the days to come. This is our private time together. I will make this same promise to you every night to keep you safe. I will tell you how much I want you and how I can't wait to meet you. I love you, little one, more than anything—and I really do. Good night, little one. My hand is on my stomach, and I am smiling as I drift off to sleep.

The next morning he says, for the family's sake, let's not bring it up when we go visit for dinner next week, OK? Really? I don't get to act excited—I don't get to talk about the one thing on my mind all day long? I don't get to even mention it. Cause it will be hard on them. Are you kidding me? That is crazy. That is absolutely, unequivocally crazy. I feel so alone and the distance between my husband and me is expanding. This is supposed to be the happiest time in a couple's life. This is supposed to bring us closer and yet I feel farther apart. I am feeling angry at him. Angry at him for not thinking about it. Angry at him for acting like it wasn't real. Angry at him for thinking about his family's feelings over mine. Angry for him not believing. Just angry at him for not acknowledging how angry and alone I feel.

We arrive at the dinner with his family, and I put on a fake smile. Everything is great—thanks for asking. Even though you didn't. I will just sit quiet, and I won't say anything. Don't yell at them or engage them and don't bring it up. Oh, great—they are talking about his brother's baby. He is walking now, and you have pictures! Sure, he is a big boy. Oh, he is cute. Everyone gathers around and comments on how cute he is, and it hurts. Don't get me wrong—I am happy for him, and the boy is super cute. However, it is a painful reminder for me. I tune back into the conversation as they proclaim excitedly that he is growing so fast. You know what else is growing fast? This baby inside of me. But don't worry—I won't bring it up.

I make some excuse to walk away from the table and am completely lost in my own thoughts. He is so cute with his big smile, round face, and blue eyes. I wonder what my baby will look like. Will it be a boy? Will he have that cute blonde hair and that cute dimple smile and those blue eyes? Wonder what he will look like? What? Do you say something? Oh, yes, he is getting big, and he looks like his father. So cute. I want to be happy for them and share in their joy. It just hurts. It is a five-by-seven glossy reminder of that fact that his baby is growing up and mine never got the chance.

We were pregnant at the same time as his brother. How could I not think if we had had a boy and how he would be getting so big? We named him Matthew. I pictured him with cherub cheeks and blonde hair and the cutest little nose. That was a thing. There are cute noses like mine (little pig nose with a round bulb at the end of it). I was not bragging about my nose but comparing it to the crooked hook noses in his family. You obsess about those things. Even on this cute little boy, his nose looked fine. I glanced at my husband and looked at this nose. It was like a hook—long and pointy. Could you picture a baby with that nose? Yeesh!! I wondered what Matthew would have been like as I listened to the stories of how his cousin was trying to walk.

My heart hurt so much. This baby was a constant reminder of what I'd lost. I was an awful person for thinking it. I certainly loved my nephew—he was super cute. I didn't mean not to fawn over him or join in on the commentary and stories and constant conversation. I really didn't—it just hurt—it was a painful reminder of my beautiful baby Matthew, whom I would never hold. It seemed like no one remembered him except me. All this chit-chat about my nephew and not a mention about the baby I was carrying now. We would just pretend they didn't exist. Ugh. I hated that. I sat down in the corner with my cup of tea. I just wanted to be alone in my sadness and my happiness. *Hey, little one. Do you like peppermint tea?*

No, thank you—I don't want coffee after supper.

But you always have coffee.

Well, I can't tonight because I am pregnant. I cannot say that. I cannot tell them that I am thinking about the health of my unborn child and avoiding all potential risks to the pregnancy. But don't worry, I won't bring it up and I won't talk about it. I won't think about the fact that I haven't had coffee or any type of caffeine or sugar in three months. But it's OK, because it isn't even a sacrifice for this little one. OMG—it is the twelve-week mark. It is three months! We made it. Umm. No, I am not smiling for anything—I am just trying something new with the tea—peppermint will be fine, thanks. Sipping my tea—I am thinking about the book I was reading about herbs and raspberry causing bleeding, so not that. Peppermint—what did it say about peppermint? I stare down into my cup. Oh, God, was it something bad for the baby? No, no. It is relaxing—it was relaxing—OK, good—breathe—great for stress. Yup, no potential harm for the baby. It relaxes the nervous system. Yep—this tea is good.

As much as I tried to hide from any type of conversation, I was failing. Yep, I was reading a book about herbs and their properties. Every herb has a healing property or is used for something. Plus, I wanted to know if anything I ate would cause another miscarriage. *Nope, I didn't say that aloud. Just reading—yep, I love to read about everything. Don't know why that is funny. Bookworm? Yep, been called that many times before. Funny, sounds just as judgemental, as it did when my mom said it. Don't know why you need to read so much. I enjoy it. Nothing else. Hahaha nope! Ugh.*

I glanced over at my husband and wondered when we could make our escape. He looked like he was enjoying himself—laughing and chatting—and he did not seem ready to leave. I was so very tired. I could just fall asleep anywhere those days. I swore I could sleep all day. That was normal for this time in pregnancy. Only what was normal about it? I couldn't talk about it—couldn't mention it. I just pretended it didn't exist and I was not exhausted. Everyone knew I was pregnant, and they just pretended I wasn't. *Oh, what? Sorry? I look tired. Well, I am pregnant. Gasp. Oh, no! I said that out loud. Yes, dear, we know. Can I get you anything else? I am going to put out some sweets for everyone.*

Oh—well, that lasted two seconds. Let's continue to pretend I am not pregnant. No *How are you feeling?* No *Rest, dear, it will pass.* Nope—just a *Let's pretend it doesn't exist.* Ugh. Torture. Utter torture. At least they will just ignore me for the rest of the night. Don't want to talk to me about my pregnancy? Nope. Too uncomfortable for you? Aw, sorry my losses are so commonplace that you just pretend they don't even exist. I am so angry—you should be happy for us., you *should be congratulating us. No thanks, I don't want any sweets—watching what I eat—oh, for no reason. My smile says you know why, but since you don't want to talk about it, you will just mention how skinny I am and walk away. Lucky her—no babies—that is why she has such a great figure. What? Are you kidding me? Did you just say that to me? No babies??? I was pregnant. I do want babies—I really do. How could you be so insensitive to say that to me? How could you be so clueless as to how hurtful that really is? I really hate these dinners. They just make me feel less of a woman—less of a wife. Yep, he would make a great father. You are right. Yep, I should give him babies. He wants a big family. Really? Yep, he has said that. And that look. Was that a look? Was that a look to say if you hadn't married her, you would have babies by now? It felt judgemental and hurtful.*

Don't worry, you will have babies one day when you are ready. Did you just say that? I look at my husband in disbelief. Are they trying to be mean? Do you believe it when they blame me? How could you? This makes me feel more terrible and even more useless. More hurt. I have had it! I stand up and declare that I am tired I want to go home. I know you don't want to, but I have had enough of this and just want to go home and cry in peace. But it won't be five more minutes, it will be another hour or so, and I cannot take one more minute of this. You don't get to enjoy yourselves and not be angry or hurt or feel so useless. I sneak to the bathroom and quietly cry. I am so angry and hurt. Don't worry, little one. We will show them. I know you will be born, and they will be fawning over you and telling you how cute you are. And I won't ever tell you how your father and his stupid family acted and pretended that you didn't exist. Nope, they will just act like nothing happened and fawn over you. It won't matter how I felt because I will be the proudest mama of them all—I will say out loud, "Why, yes! They are the cutest baby of them all. And they won't dare say different because they'll know how protective I am.

Finally, we left. "You know, honey," I said as I rolled over that night in bed. "It is almost the end of three-month mark. Thought you would be happy. I didn't embarrass you. I don't care what your family thinks of me. Don't you care about our little one? Long night? Yep, it has been. Sleep well, indeed."

Then one morning as you awake, the thought hits you. We made it. We made it through these last eight weeks. We are at the end of the first trimester!! *Hey, honey! He will be excited now. I know he will. Guess what day it is? We are almost at the end of the first trimester! Do you think we can tell a few people? My brother? Your sister? Our friends? You are hesitant?! Can you just let yourself believe for a second? Did you know all the organs are developed? I mean, that has got to be a sign, right? We made it through the most complicated parts of development— brain, hands, and feet—they are mostly developed—all the organs and systems are developed. The danger of something going wrong developmentally has passed. C'mon, really? NO! I can't just put it out my mind and, NEWS FLASH, I never did not for one second. We may not be pregnant, but I am! I have thought about our little one for every second of every day. Fine. Begrudgingly, he agrees.*

We can tell people. You should call your brother, he advises. I already did. He is helping me. Never mind. Honey, you should call your sister or your mom. Oh, this is so exciting. He is calling them. This should take a while; his sister will keep him on the phone forever and so will his mom. They will just be glad that he called. We finally get to tell people—they are going to be so happy this time. They are going to know things are different this time. They will all say "congratulations—we can't wait to meet the baby. Keep us posted on how she is doing."

What? That was quick! Did you call at a bad time? No way the conversation was that short. What did they say? That's great and take care. WHAT? That's great? Take care? Let's contain our excitement. Then what he said next shocked me: *You can't blame them, hon. You don't have the greatest history—you can't blame them for being skeptical. What? Did you just say that? Yes, I can—I blame them. I hate that they are just expecting me to lose another one. It isn't a set of keys—I am not the person who keeps losing all these keys. I am mother carrying a baby! And you just expect them to die and that is what we are going with?* He snaps at me in frustration *"What do you want me from me, hon? You really can't blame them for thinking that."* Yes. Yes, I can. You are the one person who I can count on to believe.

The day came when we decided to tell our friends. They would be excited for me. Friends are always supportive and encouraging. I was so excited; it would be so great to finally have someone to chat with. But we made this big announcement in front of them and there was no celebration. *Hopeful—did she say hopeful? You meant to say you are excited that we are pregnant. Right? Yeah, but hopeful, and try not to think about it. I am stunned. Shocked.*

I wanted to scream that I thought about it every second of every day and that suggesting otherwise was incredibly naïve. But instead, I smiled weakly, and thought: is it really that easy for everyone? I wondered, when people make comments like: *Well, just because it is in there doesn't mean it will come out.* And *just be realistic.* If only they knew how incredibly hurtful it was and that it was not at all helpful. You become numb with the unwitting comments. You just cannot believe the responses. Thank goodness they have never experienced this tragedy, that they don't know the actual hurt they are causing you. Besides the hurt, you also feel cheated. You are cheated out of the epic movie and TV scenes of the pregnancy announcement. *What happened to the congratulations, we are so happy for you, you are going to be a great mom, this baby is so lucky?*

The comments are the same at six weeks, twelve weeks, and even later. I understand people don't know what to say, but the hurt is the same. *I am at almost sixteen weeks and that is what you say?* At that point, you have read so much information about the baby's development. They are fully developed, including their hearing. They can hear these comments! You suddenly feel sad and try to comfort the little one inside you. *I hope you don't understand them, little one.*

I am tired, honey, and I want to go home—nope, not in five minutes. Now. How are you not mad? How are you not angry? Why do we call these people friends? What, you understand how they feel? How about how I feel? How about how you feel? Why aren't you mad? Why aren't you insulted? Why does it feel like there is an us and them and you are on the side of them? Don't bother coming to the doctor's appointment this week. Nope, I am good. Don't bother. It's starting to feel like you don't believe our baby is going to be born. We are sixteen weeks along. But, hey, continue not to think about it. Ugh, why are we fighting so much? Why am I so angry? Why isn't he?

The doctor's appointment is tomorrow. I am excited they are going to book an ultrasound and I might finally get to see the baby. They don't book ultrasounds when you are "high-risk," and you certainly don't get to see them or take home that ultrasound picture to hang on the fridge. *This time, they will let me see it. After all, I am over four months along. They need to let me see this one—they must let me see this time. Oh, little one, I can't wait to see you—in blurry grey and white but I will be able to see your head. After all these days and nights of chatting to you, I will get to see you move around.* That night, I went to sleep with my hand on my stomach, saying, "Good night, little one" and telling them about how I would get to see them tomorrow. *Just think, we made it through another day. I love you, little one.*

Every time that it happened, I just had to keep telling myself this time would result in a baby.

Chapter 5

My Hardest Loss—Second Trimester

THE BEGINNING OF YOUR SECOND TRIMESTER IS A TIME FOR celebration, especially after you have experienced a miscarriage. This is where you can feel like you can breathe again. Since most miscarriages occur in the first trimester, making it to the second trimester is a huge relief for couples. It is when you feel safe telling people. You feel like you can announce it to the world. After all, even if you had a miscarriage in the first trimester, this is different—it is the second trimester.

You have passed a huge hurdle! You are starting to show more than the bulge of the first trimester—this is looking like the start of a cute baby bump. It is your billboard to the world: yes, we have made it and we are pregnant. After experiencing a miscarriage, you still feel a level of apprehension and downright fear at times, and that is expected. Even past the scary first trimester, trepidation is expected.

When you start announcing it to your friends, you might still receive insensitive responses, even from the most unexpected people. It seems like a simple congratulations may just be beyond the capacity of most of your friends and family group. They may feel the need to remind you of the previous miscarriage and caution you not to be too excited as things happen. At these comments, I was quite surprised, because they had previously dismissed my miscarriage so quickly and never wanted to talk about it. Then they bring it up as if you could have forgotten. They didn't want to talk about it before and now they are full of advice and caution. Did I mention a huge part of this experience is the ability not to respond and to fight the urge to slap people? All kidding aside, it is one of the toughest things to endure. I mean, from your single friends—a myriad "Oh, wow, you are trying again" to "Do you think it will work this time?" is mildly expected. But the completely insensitive, most hurtful comments that are going to blindside you will come from your family, who should be your greatest source of support. These comments will be the hardest to ignore and, if you are like me, will be the endless source of private car rants. Just know that you are not alone in these feelings.

After your announcements are done and you are settled into the seventeenth or eighteenth week, you feel pretty darn good. You start to pick out maternity clothes or at least go to a few shops and think about it. Don't expect your friend group to offer to join you as they might still be expecting to see what happens—whether they admit it or not. As you have realized by this point in your experiences, your partner becomes your sole source of support.

Every day you allow yourself to believe a little more and be happy a little more. You let your guard down—just a little. You almost don't expect it anymore. But for me, this worry never went away. I remember asking my mom when you stop worrying about your baby—when it is born, after the first year, when they start school or college, or what—and my mother said it's when you draw your last breath. OK, but I just had to get through the pregnancy, and I would worry less (another story for another time—hint, you worry just as much, if not more).

This time in the pregnancy is filled with tangible proof of your baby. You are feeling your baby kick and so is your partner. You have always talked to them, but now your partner is talking to them—saying good night and good morning. It is truly wonderful. I remember changing the radio station because my baby moved more when a good song was on. It was a great time—we were having a dance party. You start saying things like, "Baby wants some pizza tonight," or "Baby is asking for ice cream," and your partner justifies bringing home certain foods for the baby. I knew they wanted to try this cake, so I got it. The books tell you the second trimester is one of the best times of the pregnancy. Any nausea or tiredness of the first trimester has passed. You have a surge of energy, and your hormone surges are making you extremely happy. This may result in inconsolable ugly crying for no reason or in response to commercials with babies.

It is the time when you feel the best during your pregnancy. This is before the final trimester, when you're huge as a house and not able to see your toes. It's still before the baby starts to squeeze your organs and insides and before the dashes to the bathroom with random pee dribbles, which are always frustrating—mainly because you cannot dash and make it in time.

The second trimester is the best time physically in your pregnancy. It is your time to enjoy being pregnant and to show it off. Relish in your friends' compliments and mentions of your glow and questions about how the baby is.

So, when one morning I unexpectedly started to get that heavy feeling in my stomach like a rock, I knew it wasn't good. You just know. I panicked and went immediately home to lie down. *Nothing is wrong—I am just tired—must be touch of the flu.* I didn't call anyone to ask for advice because I had learned that their opinions were not helpful or comforting. I was panicking, and I was having a hard time breathing. It felt like something was wrong.

As my husband arrived home and saw me lying down, he looked at me with immediate panic. A side effect of miscarriages is that you are both on the brink of panicking. You are robbed of the complete blissfulness and peace that most woman experience at this stage. We needed to go to the doctor. Something was wrong. *Honey, please trust me.* We got into the car to drive to emergency. What was wrong—what happened? I couldn't say it—I couldn't tell him. I couldn't say it because I didn't want it to be true. *Please, just drive. There is a pressure and I started bleeding*, I said quietly, just minutes from the emergency room. *I am sure it is fine—I just need to check it out.*

After hours of waiting in the emergency room and finally seeing a doctor, they did an ultrasound and told us to go home. If the bleeding gets heavier, they told us, come back, or call your doctor. This is where you tell yourself that everything is fine and if it wasn't, the hospital would have known. They would never have let you go home if there was a chance that something would happen to the baby. Complications in the second trimester are rare, the nurse assured me. "Complications" is hospital-speak for the danger of losing your baby. That night, I couldn't sleep and all I could do was keep talking to my baby and promising that everything would be OK. *We made it this far, didn't we? We are survivors and we are going to make it. We are almost two-thirds of the way. Hang in there, my sweet baby.*

By the next night, the bleeding was worse, the pain was worse, and we headed back to the hospital. I kept chanting the constant mantra that everything was going to be OK. *I just bought my first maternity top this week—this cannot be happening.* All these thoughts were flooding my mind as we arrived at the hospital. I was not sure how much time passed as I lay on a bed in the emergency room. A nurse was trying to put an IV in my hand and could not seem to find a vein. She was poking me over and over and kept saying how small my veins were. Eventually, she got another nurse. The second nurse put the IV in the side of my wrist, which was painful. My hand was very cold and there was a sharp pain where the IV was inserted.

I asked the nurse what was going on and she said I was pale and dehydrated. A doctor would be in soon, she said. *Please, is my baby OK?* She just smiled and left. I could feel the tears roll down my face as I stared at my husband. *It has got to be OK, right?* He looked pale and very frightened. The doctor came in and said that my blood pressure was low, so they were going to do an ultrasound to make sure everything was all right with the baby.

In typical fashion, the ride to the ultrasound was quiet and they didn't let me see the screen during the ultrasound. I really wanted to see if my baby was OK, I told them, but that comment was ignored. The tech was looking at the screen very intently and I was looking for any indication on her face to let me know it was OK. The whole time I was praying and panicking and quietly crying. My husband wasn't allowed in the room, and I felt very alone and scared.

After the ultrasound, they brought me to a room and my husband was there. *What happened? Did they say anything? No—I don't know.* My husband informed me that he must leave as it was the weekend of his cousin's wedding and all his family had flown in for this event. *Please call my brother so I have someone here with me*, I said. *And I think you should tell your family. I cannot possibly tell them what is going on*, he said. *Well, maybe they will want to be here with me*, I responded. He looked at me like he didn't want to cause any issues. *Let's not take away from her day*, he said as he quickly left the room. Anger rose inside me and quickly faded into sadness and fear.

I felt so alone and scared. I was feeling so anxious and panicked. I was trying to take deep breaths and tell myself I needed to brave for my baby. I kept saying softly that it was going to be OK, little one. *Everything is going to be OK. I promise. We will make it through this. We are survivors.* Only it didn't feel OK. There was a pressure in my stomach. I was trying to feel my baby kick or move, and I didn't feel anything.

Since I had no concept of time at this point, I am not sure how long I was lying there. A nurse came in and changed the IV bag and added another one without saying a word. She left as quickly as she came in. A doctor finally came in and stated that they could not find a heartbeat. My heart was beating so loudly in my ears, and he continued to talk. "What?" I said. "Are you sure?" At that moment, I was stunned. I couldn't believe it and I wouldn't believe it. "Am I going to lose the baby?" The doctor simply said that the baby was not viable and there was no heartbeat. But I was eighteen weeks along and had just bought my first maternity top. He continued to say that they were going to wait to see if I start to expel it on my own over the next few hours. If not, then they would explore other options. It sounded as if he was talking in a tunnel and was a million miles away. I could barely hear him. All I could hear was the pounding of my heartbeat. I was breathing deeply by then and apparently hyperventilating because the next thing I remember is a nurse putting oxygen on me. "Nice, slow breaths," she said. I was crying and looking at her like she was an alien and speaking another language. "Continue to monitor her vitals and keep me posted," the doctor said, and left my room. The nurse placed a monitor on my hand and left quickly after that.

I was alone again. *What did he say? The baby's heart is not beating and is not viable. You mean dead? My baby is dead and is inside me! This cannot be happening. This isn't real. This must be a dream.* My brother entered the room, and he was normally a very calm and stoic individual. He saw me in the hospital many times when I was younger, and he always made me feel better. He doesn't panic and is a very calm presence. He always made me feel better and would even make me laugh. But now he was visibly shaken, and I had not seen him like that before.

"How are you?" he asked quietly.

"They told me that my baby's heartbeat has stopped, and it is no longer viable. My baby is dead!" I started to cry, which only made him more uncomfortable.

"Please stay with me. Please don't leave me. I can't do this. I don't want to be alone. I am so scared."

"I am not leaving," he declared. "You are the strongest person I know, and you can get through this. You are not alone. I am here."

I felt slightly better. My hand was on my stomach, and I said I couldn't feel the baby move anymore and started to cry harder.

"What are they going to do?" he asked.

"They want me to expel it on my own."

"What?" he said. "That sounds crazy." I smiled a little.

I wasn't sure how much time had passed, and it felt like I was frozen in time. I was still bleeding heavily and the pressure in my stomach had continued to increase. The doctor checked on me and asked how I was feeling. I stared at him, and I knew he meant *Has something happened to help expel the baby?* I asked him what to expect and he said they were going to continue to give me fluids and see what happened over the next twelve hours before considering other options. *What? What does that mean?* "The best-case scenario would be for you to pass the fetus on your own and then we can do a complete D&C after." The *best case?* That isn't *my* best-case scenario—you could tell me you were wrong, and the heartbeat was OK. This wasn't best case. There wasn't an option for a viable fetus at that point. That is really a medical way of saying that you have a dead baby inside of you. That, after months of talking to and planning your life around this baby, it is dead, and they will leave it inside you to see if you start to expel it naturally. Seriously, can you be more callous?

The bleeding continued through the night and the cramping got more intense and, at some point, they decided I was losing so much blood that they gave me a transfusion. I had several tubes in me now—monitors and IV and other tubes that I had no idea about. *You must push out the fetus just like a live birth.* Nice terms, eh? I can't explain how incredibly numb I felt at this point. There are just no words to describe this experience. It was long and painful and soul wrenching.

Afterward, I was taken to the operating room so they could perform a D&C. This is basically a procedure to dilate and scrape out the remains from your womb. As much as they assure you it is a common procedure and practically day surgery, I can assure you, it is most certainly not simple. Afterward, they pumped some more IV fluids and antibiotics because infection is the biggest concern at this point, they explained. I can assure you; it was not my biggest concern. The loss of my baby was and knowing that it was dead inside of me. I don't think I will ever forget that feeling.

After they pumped more fluids in me and monitored me throughout the night, I was told I would be released the next morning. They would perform an autopsy on the fetus and let me know if they found anything. I was feeling so incredibly weak, both physically and emotionally drained. Had I heard that right? I was well enough to go home. I felt like I had been punched in the stomach and the cramping and soreness had not receded at all. But walking out of that hospital the next morning—well, shuffling out of the hospital down the hallways with pregnant ladies all around—was one of the loneliest feelings in the world. I was empty. I was just supposed to go home and forget about this. I shuffled to the car and sat silently all the way home.

Chapter 6
Third-Trimester Complications

AFTER MANY MISCARRIAGES, I COULDN'T BELIEVE I HAD MADE it to the third trimester with this pregnancy. This was the first time we made it to the third trimester. The next morning was like every other morning. I put my hand on my stomach and say good morning to my little one. I felt great and happy. I should be happy—I was starting to really show. I should be showing—I was almost twenty-five weeks. This was the start of the third trimester. We had made it!!

The doctor said the baby was healthy and the heartbeat was strong. I was feeling great—no pains, no more nausea, and no more mind-numbing exhaustion. I was feeling energized. Pretty soon, people would be asking me when I was due. I looked in the bathroom mirror and there was a giant smile on my face. I was so happy—I still checked the tissue when I wiped but the constant panic wasn't there. I didn't expect to see the blood anymore—well, not as much. I would have to start thinking about shopping for maternity clothes. After my second term loss, I didn't want to go maternity clothes shopping until the last possible second. My husband would soon start talking about the baby non-stop and we could plan and dream together. This was going to be a great day.

After lunch there was a dull ache in my lower stomach. Panic set in. *I shouldn't have come to work today. Stop it. Don't worry. It is probably something you ate. Maybe you need a bowel movement. Your baby is fine, and you are fine. Breathe. Remember what the doctor said—everything was fine.* When I met my husband after work we were going to walk through the mall and look at the maternity shop. Well, maybe just glance at the rack at the beginning of the store. Not actually go in. Maybe just for a second go in and look at the tops on the rack. Just breathe and get through this day. *It is OK, little one. It is nothing. I put your hand on my stomach. Like holding my stomach means holding them—protecting them.*

It is around four o'clock and I am almost at the end of the workday. I went to the washroom. The ache was still there—it felt like a rock. I just needed to go to the washroom and then I would feel better. *But don't strain or push. Just wipe and look—NO!!! There is some blood—it is dark—maybe it isn't blood. I wipe again. Oh, God, there is more! No!! I panic and a wave of heat goes over my body. NO!! it can't be—the doctor said everything looked great! Should I call her? No—it is Friday at 4 p.m., and there is no way I can get in. There is nothing to worry about. I am too far along; this cannot be happening. Just breathe. Breathe. OK, think—what did you eat? What did you do? You walked around at lunch in the mall—was that too much? I was tired and I thought it would wake me up. Maybe I should have just rested. I shouldn't have gone for that walk. OH, GOD, what did I do? This is my fault. No—don't think that. Don't go to worst-case scenario. Remain positive for the little one. Don't worry, little one—Oh, God, they can feel my emotions—I read that in the book. I am not panicking, little one—I promise. It is going to be OK. I will protect you. I won't let anything happen to you. I promise. Oh, sweet Jesus in heaven. Guardian angels, please protect my little one—please don't let anything happen to them.*

There is knock on the bathroom door – it is my co-worker. Yes, I am OK. I will be right out. OK—breathe. Pull yourself together. Am I OK? Yes, of course. I am fine. She looks at me with concern. Is everything OK with-you-know? as she looks at my stomach. That is what people do when they know you have had miscarriages, they don't refer to your baby or pregnancy directly. With my baby? Of course, I snapped. Why wouldn't it be—why would you think something was wrong? I was practically screaming at her. I breathed as she looked back at me, shocked and stunned. "I think I have the flu," I tell her. "I am just going to gather my stuff and leave early. I don't feel well—sorry I yelled at you." *Sorry not sorry, I think—you were the one thinking something was wrong with my baby.*

I quietly gathered my things and walked out—apologizing for the early exit. *Why am I apologizing to them?* "See you tomorrow," they say. Because God forbid, I take a day off. Three years and I hadn't even taken a sick day. Not one. Just two days off when I lost the last one. I worked so many long hours of overtime without getting paid, and I was always the last one to leave the office. *But, yeah, everything is fine—see you tomorrow.* I walked over to the store where my husband worked and told him I wasn't feeling well. "I will be off in fifteen minutes," he said. "Is everything OK? he said, looking at my stomach. I couldn't admit it—I wouldn't admit it. *I am just not feeling well.* Since we only had one car, I was stuck sitting in there, trying not to panic—trying not to cry. *It will be OK—everything is OK. Just go home and rest—put your feet up—with the pillows under your knees—elevate them and everything will be fine.* I breathe in and out slowly and hold my stomach. *The pain is going away, right? It feels less heavy, right? Oh, God, is that wetness you feel? Please, no! No, it isn't. You are just panicking—breathe. Breathe. They can feel emotions—don't worry, little one, I am calm—we are going to be OK; I promise you. Remember, I promised I would take care of you, and you are going to be just fine. Promise me you will hang on—promise me you will be OK. It is just us. Promise me. Please be OK. Please be OK.* It is my mantra. It felt like hours passed. Where was he? He had promised. He finally got in the car. "Are you OK?"

"Can you just drive?" I snapped. *Why does everyone assume it is not OK? Why does everyone think I will just lose the baby? Oh, God. Stop thinking like that—just breathe—you will be home soon. Put your feet up.*

The baby wasn't due until the first week of July and it was only April. I couldn't believe this was happening again—the bleeding. I had been lying there with my legs on the pillows for two days. Not wanting to go to the bathroom because I would see the blood again and that feeling of utter panic would consume me. That wave of sadness and panic and utter desperation. What did the doctor say again? If the bleeding got worse or if it didn't stop, then go to emergency. It wasn't stopping, but was it worse? It was hard to tell. The sight of the blood every time I went to the washroom—was it more? I couldn't tell. It seemed like a lot. It should have stopped.

Then I started to torture myself with the familiar debate. Should we go to emergency? Should we try to call the doctor? It was too late to call the doctor. I didn't want to go to emergency because, when I go there, I lose the baby and they never, ever do anything to stop it. *There is nothing we can do*, they always say. *These things happen. If there is nothing you can do, then why do I go to emergency and sit there in public for hours, hoping and wanting you to do something? I feel so desperate, and they keep telling me there is nothing we can do. These things happen. Like what? When you get rain, and the weatherman didn't predict it—then you can say "these things happen," but you do absolutely nothing while someone loses a baby and yes, it is a baby. Then that isn't the time when you say those things happen.* It is not a thing *that happens.* It is a horrible and devasting event. You can't cry or scream at them because that isn't acceptable. *Do you need something to calm you down? Yes, I do. Can you save my baby? But, no, I don't need a sedative or a muscle relaxant.* But what if they can actually do something—what if this is the one time that they tell you that if you would have just come in earlier, we could have done something? You can't live with that regret. That you didn't go into the hospital earlier and that they could have done something. You must put yourself through that excruciating experience for that glimmer of hope. Even though the dozen times before they couldn't do anything, maybe this time will be different. You can't chance it.

"We are going to the hospital," I announced.

He gave me that look—*No, don't you dare look at me like that. Don't you dare look at me like I am losing this baby—I am not. Yes, we are going because maybe this time— they can help. I don't know what they can do but maybe this time they can do something. I can't just make promises that everything is going to be OK and not do anything.* So, I bundled up and put a pad on and prayed that when I put my head back on that pillow that night that I could keep my promise. That I will have kept my baby safe.

We walked into the emergency room. I was twenty-five weeks pregnant, and I was experiencing bleeding. For how long? For about forty-nine hours. How much? Rivers and rivers of it. It seemed that way. Um. Spotting? No, more than spotting. This is so humiliating. More than a cup. I didn't squeeze it into a measuring cup. A cup? More than a cup since forty-nine-and-a-half hours ago—yes. More than a cup in the last hour—no. My doctor said if it didn't stop or if it got worse to come in. *It didn't stop. Is it worse? It feels worse. It feels like it is more but every time I wipe myself, I want to see nothing, but I see a streak of bright red blood. Is there pain? Yes—a dull cramp-like heaviness. No. Not sharp pain. There was only a sharp pain with the ectopic pregnancy, and this isn't ectopic. Is this your first pregnancy? No. Have you miscarried before? Yes. But I am not this time. This is me being pregnant and encountering difficulties—don't assume it is a miscarriage. How many miscarriages? About twelve or so. Yes, I remember the exact number. Can you be more specific? Are you talking miscarriages over three months or just ones that were under the eight-week mark? The look. That shocked, familiar look. I see that you have been hospitalized before for miscarriages.*

Yes, I have.

For how many miscarriages were you hospitalized?

Does it matter? Is this really what we want to focus on now? Can't you see that I am freaking out? Don't you understand I made a promise? I need to sit down—I feel weak. You talk to them—I am going to sit down. I hear them asking faintly: Is your wife going to be OK?

Well, let's see, we are in the emergency room, and I am praying this time that all these stupid tortuous questions and the long, agonizing wait in the examination area will not be a complete waste of time. Just smile and say she's fine. That is what you must do. Otherwise, they think you are crazy to be so emotional, like somehow being upset caused this to happen. Oh, wait—do you think the nurse won't say it this time—you know being upset isn't helping the baby? I mean, seriously, can we just think about that statement and the fact that you said it out loud to me for a second? Can you just for a second think about how utterly ridiculous that sounds? Of course, I am upset—my baby is in danger, and I can't help them, I start to cry. I notice the judging sideways looks as they quietly talk to my husband. I am the one carrying the baby—I am one holding my breath for a miracle this time. But let's talk about it like it doesn't involve me at all.

They discreetly took me to an examination room and a doctor entered and started asking the same questions. *When did the bleeding start—about fifty hours ago. Would you say it is more than spotting or does it fill a pad and how often? Would you say every hour? How would you know, Doc? Have you worn a pad—do you know about flow? Do you know the difference between a super-maxi and a maxi (because those are pretty important differences)? We are going to send you down for an ultrasound. I can feel the baby kick. Did I tell you that? We just want to take a look and see what is going on—OK? What?? Do you know how stupid that sounds—you want to take a look at the baby? I am bleeding, that is what is going on, and I am praying my little one is OK. But, sure, if it makes you feel better, Doc.*

Another two hours passed, and a young orderly came up with a wheelchair. *You are scheduled for an ultrasound.* "He is coming with me," I declared, as I pointed to my husband. The orderly looked nervous like he was about to protest. "He is my husband, and he is coming with me. It is not better if he waits here. But it is better for me if he comes. I am not asking you; I am *telling* you." *I have been here for six hours, and I am freaking out and I need him to tell me it is going to be OK. I just need to hear that. I need to cling to that tiny piece of hope, so I don't completely shatter apart at the possibility of losing another baby.* The young orderly looked just as uncomfortable and awkward as my husband at this point. I simply did not care as it wasn't about them. We walked in silence as I listened to the familiar sound of the wheelchair on the floor and the banging of the chair as we got on the elevator. *Honestly, could you have made that more graceful? Little one—you are going to be all right. Do you hear me? Don't panic. All this banging around and noise—it is unfamiliar noise—it is scary, whirring, and hushed murmuring noises. But don't worry, it will be OK—please, hang on. We will get through this together.* And we are parking, and he is leaving. Without a word he just walks away and slams my chart on the counter. Not a word. Not a single word from anyone.

I get this is your job and lots of things happen in the hospital, but people deserve some acknowledgement, some conversation, anything. This feels like the worst moment right now and I am so scared, and no one is saying anything to me. After a bit—I am assuming a half hour or so—I started to shiver. The gown and the little blanket, which clearly was too small for any person, was barely covering my lap. My legs looked blue. Thank God, they let me keep my socks. I looked down and stared blankly at my feet scrunched up on the steel foot pads. This would be different this time. Everything was going to be OK. They were going to say, "Thank God you came in and that was so smart of you. What a great mom you are going to make."

What? Yes, that is my name tag.

They wheeled me into the ultrasound room. I laid down on the table and put the cover over me. The tech left. I knew the drill—this was all too familiar.

I hate ultrasounds. In high-risk pregnancies, they only do them when there is something wrong. There was a fear that the radiation was harmful to the fetus. My friend had one and they showed them the picture and they got to take it home. They have it on the fridge. It looks like an ink blot, but they show everyone, and they get to be excited. With "high-risk" pregnancies, you don't get a picture. Why? Has someone used it as evidence of a perfectly healthy baby and sued you? *Look, Your Honour, this clearly shows a happy and healthy baby—I think that is the head and it looks like a perfectly good head.* Nothing wrong there. So, what happened?

The tech silently walked in and sat down. She said quietly, "This might be a little cold." Classic understatement. It felt like she was drizzling liquid ice on my body. She purposely turned the monitor away so I couldn't see it. Click, click. Click. "Can you see anything?" I asked.

"I am just taking the pictures, I can't say."

Click-click-click, a few dozen more times in silence. I looked, panicked, at my husband and struggled a smile—it-is-going-to-be-OK-this-time kind of a smile. But he just looked blankly at me. Was he even trying to see the screen? No? Why not? *You can see the baby and tell me it looks like a perfectly fine head.* "I am done," she declared. "Just wait and I will check to make sure the pictures are fine." She left.

"Well, did you see anything?"

"No, I couldn't. I was over here."

"OK, but this is a super small room, and she turned the screen away from me so you could have tried to look."

Why? I was looking for a tiny shred of hope. *I saw the head—it looked fine—it was moving. Anything.* I was not going to record it and present it in a court of law. *Just lie to me.* I looked at him with such exasperation, like he should be feeling just as panicked and hopeless as I did. I was searching for that tiny bit of hope, so the floor didn't open up and swallow me.

"Well??" I say.

"Well, what? She will be back, and everything will be fine."

Ugh, why do I find that so incredibly infuriating? I just want to know that you are panicking too or that you care? I stared at the wall, unable to speak. *Don't cry. Please don't cry—just hold it together. It will be OK, little one.*

She came back in and declared that the pictures were fine. "Someone will be along to bring you back to the exam room."

"Is the baby OK?" I asked, and she replied that the doctor would tell us the results.

"I know, but does he look OK?"

She just smiled and left. *Was that a sympathy smile? Was that a don't-worry smile? Did you see that? What do you think?*

I didn't see anything—I don't know—let's just wait.

Ugh. Still desperately looking for tiny glimmer of hope to hang onto, but, sure, let's sit and wait for another few hours for the vague comments that we are so used to hearing.

We were back waiting in the exam room for what seemed like hours. I was so cold!!! I really didn't know why they let me sit there in that stupid little gown. I was practically an ice cube at this point. "I am cold," I told him.

"It isn't cold here," he said, but he was bundled up in his winter coat and sweatshirt and jeans.

"Oh, really? Not even a little?"

"Nope, I am fine."

"Can I have my coat?"

"Just wait for the doctor and then we can get dressed."

I felt all my emotions about to explode on him. Unfair? Absolutely. But excuse me! *We can get dressed. You are dressed and bundled in your clothes, and I am in this cloth gown. I have told you that I am freezing, so it isn't* we *who will be getting dressed! It is* me *not dressed and freezing. Can I just have my coat?*

The doctor walked in. *Everything looks fine. Go home and monitor the bleeding and call your doctor on Monday.*

What is causing the bleeding?

Nothing we can find. Everything looks OK. If the bleeding stops, then it will be fine; if it continues through the weekend, call your doctor.

But isn't there anything you can do? To help stop the bleeding.

He turned and talked to my husband again. He politely thanked the doctor for his time and help and the doctor left the room.

I stared at him, feeling another rant building up. *What was that? What? You were thanking him for what, exactly? He didn't tell us anything and we didn't even get to see the slides. The just-go-home-and-wait speech. We had a chance for some answers this time. Is that enough for you, because it isn't for me. I feel just as panicked and freaked out as I did fourteen hours ago.*

"Please get dressed so we can go home."

The Empty Crib

"Can you help me?"

"Why?"

"Because I am afraid to bend down because it might cause more bleeding or hurt the baby. Because I have been afraid to move and breathe for the past three days and not to mention I am freezing and cannot feel my hands or legs or any of my limbs. I still feel the heavy feeling in my stomach, and it has lasted for three days, and I don't want to lose this baby!"

The drive home was silent. I was silently crying, and I just wanted him to say something to comfort me. He knew everything he said would be met with another rant, but I still just needed him to tell me he believed the baby was fine.

We got home and I crawled into bed with my legs once again over the pillow at the end. I put my hand on my stomach. *Hey, little one, it is going to be OK. I know it is—please hang in there. There is nothing wrong. Don't worry. I promise—I got you. I love you, little one.* I silently prayed, promising I would do anything to make sure this baby was OK. *Please, God, please let them be OK. Please.*

I lay in bed for two days, only getting up only when necessary to go to the washroom. Wiping and inspecting the colour, the amount—something that would give me a clue. My husband called the doctor, and she could see us Monday afternoon. She said that if we stopped bleeding, we didn't have to come in. I looked perplexed at this comment. *Don't worry, little one, you are not alone, and I believe everything will be fine. I have tons of optimism and hope and I believe, even if no one else does.*

Chapter 7
The Impossible Choice

MONDAY AFTERNOON ARRIVED, AND IT FELT ALL TOO FAMILIAR. I was sitting in my OB's patient room waiting for her to come in. I was almost eight months along and this was the longest I had been pregnant. I am sitting there on the table as the doctor goes over the chart and slides from the ultrasound. In silence. In deaf-defying silence. Then she said that everything looked fine, but that we must consider the situation.

The "situation"? What do you mean?

If everything looks fine and the baby is OK, then there is no situation. You have been bleeding for almost a week (five days—not really a week) *and it hasn't stopped. It hasn't gotten any worse and there have been no clots.* I was convinced that she needed more information.

"That is a good sign, right?"

She was quiet. Then she said that we must consider that maybe we didn't know what effect this had on the fetus. Bleeding at this stage wasn't a good indication of the status of the pregnancy. I was completely numb. "What about another ultrasound or an amniocentesis? I know it isn't recommended on 'high-risk' pregnancies, but if we are really worried about the state of the baby . . ."

Obviously, she hadn't finished her thought, so she continued without acknowledging my comments. "We need to consider the effect on your health and your capacity to carry a child full term."

I was stunned. *What?*

"You have had numerous pregnancies and miscarriages and we have to consider your health at this point and your mental state."

Pardon me?

"The doctor noted that you were very upset in the emergency room."

"Isn't that expected?" I countered. "Of course, I was upset. What does my mental state have to do with anything? Are you acknowledging for once that this is difficult on me? Of course, it is hard. I lost my babies."

She then looked at my husband. "We have to consider what is best and face some realities. I have been a high-risk obstetrician for twenty years and I must consider the number of miscarriages that your wife has had and the current risks to this pregnancy. Technically, the fetus does not appear to be in distress, but we must consider options. We have to consider that the best option may be to choose to terminate this pregnancy."

I was stunned—I just stared at her. I shouted that was my choice and not theirs—either of theirs. I was angry and they appeared to be leaving me out of this conversation.

She stopped talking to my husband and they both just stared at me—like how your parents look at you when you interrupt them. I asked her very slowly and pointedly, "Do you know if the baby is healthy?"

"Well, the fetus . . ." and I interrupted her. "No! The baby—my baby! Is the baby OK?"

She started to talk very slowly. "There is no indication at this point . . ." So, I interrupted again: *Is the baby OK? Am I losing it?* She continued: "Well, we have to consider . . ."

Answer my question: *Am I losing the baby?*

"The bleeding hasn't stopped," she announced.

Yes. I acknowledged that. *Trust me, I know. Every second since it started, I have been praying and holding my breath and telling my baby that everything was going to be OK.*

She turned to talk with my husband again. *You really should consider the options for the health of your wife. Nope—choosing to terminate this baby—not an option. There is nothing wrong with the baby. Not an option.* He carefully said that he thought we should consider this option and I shot him a look of utter betrayal and murderous rage.

Let me be clear: since it is my health and my mental state, then it is my decision. We are not discussing this further. Not for a single second more. If I miscarry, then you will have to deal with it. I am not choosing to terminate a pregnancy. If you know anything about my mental state, then you know I couldn't choose that option after what I have been through.

The doctor continued as I started to get ready to leave.

We must consider what may happen and the danger to you.

I know what it is like to lose a baby at this stage in the pregnancy.

Yes, I see that from your records.

Then trust me when I say I know completely what will happen and how it will affect me. I am not choosing to terminate.

We should discuss this further.

I interrupt: "Is there anything else you need from me today?"

"We are not done here."

"We are, Doctor. My next appointment is two weeks from tomorrow, right? I will see you then."

"If anything happens in the meantime, then go to emergency and please consider what I have said."

I stormed out of the doctor's office, completely outraged, and hurt. We didn't say anything until we got to the car.

The baby is OK. Did you hear that part? That is the news I have been waiting to hear since Friday night at emergency, which may only seem like it has been a few days ago to you but it has been an eternity for me. The baby is OK. I kept saying as a comfort to me as much as a declaration to him.

"We should consider what could happen," my husband said, and I looked at him with such shock and disbelief. "Are you kidding me? Who do you think you are talking to? For every single miscarriage, I have been through it—you haven't. For the ones I didn't call you for because I knew what was happening and couldn't bear that look of frustration and hurt in your eyes. For the few times at the hospital where I told you it was OK and not to come, that I was OK. I wasn't. I know your family was in town for that one, but I wasn't OK. The last time I lost a baby that was around this stage was inconvenient when your cousin was getting married, and your entire family flew in. I am bringing it up again. I didn't need a reminder of the days I lay there by myself alone and wishing you would come and knowing you wanted to see your family. You don't know what I went through so you don't get to decide on this, and you don't get to say that I should consider this. "

I continued my rant, and I was sure he didn't completely understand my point of view. "You chose not to think about this pregnancy and the baby. I understand that is your way of coping with everything. Maybe that detachment makes it easier for you to ask me to consider what she just said. I hope not, but I don't know. I thought of all the people in the world, *you* would understand and fight for our baby. You are supposed to want to fight for our baby. *You are the dad.*"

"I just think we should consider our options," he said meekly.

"You can think and consider all you want, but I AM NOT choosing to terminate this baby. I know better than anyone the pain of losing a baby, the pain of lying there helplessly and doing nothing as I lose another baby. As it feels like my very soul and insides are leaving me. The emptiness and the sadness that nobody wants to talk about, and nobody wants you to mention. It was only as big as a grapefruit or whatever analogy, so it is no big deal. Except it is. This is my baby, and I cannot choose to go through that willingly. I just cannot. If it happens again, then so be it. But I cannot *choose* that—do you understand? Of everything that I went through I simply cannot choose this. I would rather go through a dozen more than willingly choose to terminate a pregnancy. Do you understand? I am not strong enough to live with that choice.

"I don't know why those miscarriages happened and I know the agony of no answers. How I would go through everything I ate, everything I did, every emotion, looking for the trigger that could have possibly explained what led to it. But I cannot choose it. I understand people choose to terminate pregnancies for a lot of reasons and that is their choice and their circumstances. I offer no judgement regarding that, only love and understanding knowing that it was an impossible choice for the mother. An impossible choice that should not be judged or commented upon or mentioned by anyone.

"I will do anything for this baby. I would choose to stand on my head for the remaining weeks. I would lie in bed and minimize my breathing. I would frantically pray and plead for my baby's life every moment of my waking hours. I would do anything to keep this baby. So, to consciously choose to terminate them when I promised them every night and every morning to protect them and that it was going to be OK? I couldn't. I won't. I am not strong enough to continue after knowing I chose it. Do you want to know where my breaking point is? This is. I would never want to try again. That is final.

"Hate me if you want to, but I would hate myself more if I chose it and I would never, ever forgive you for supporting such a choice. Do you understand? I am my mother's daughter. I am crazy and stubborn, and I will stand up against the whole world for my baby. Do you understand?"

I don't know if he did or didn't—he just knew I wasn't going to budge on this. Four days later, the bleeding stopped. I was thrilled and thought this would be the end of this "option" and just knew everything was going to be fine after that point.

When we arrived at our next OB appointment, we were thrilled. How is everything? Absolutely wonderful, I exclaimed with excitement and pride with my hand on my stomach. Did you consider any more of what we talked about last time? What? The bleeding has stopped, I told her, sure she wouldn't be bringing this up if she knew.

"It could start up again and I think we need to consider . . ."

"No! We are not considering or talking about this again."

"I have been doing this for over twenty years and I only deal with high-risk pregnancies," she declared.

"I know," I acknowledged as she continued to state that there had never been a successful pregnancy with these types of complications. "It could mean permanent damage to your reproductive system if you endure another loss at this stage."

The intimidation and tension were palatable in the room. I looked at my husband, wavering in my confidence and excitement. He looked down. Oh, no! He was caving—she was winning him over. At that point, I heard my mom's voice say, *I don't care if you are the pope or the president or God Himself—this is my child!* My mom wouldn't let anyone intimidate her. She was a strong woman—she honestly didn't care if you were a priest or the prime minister (a story for another time) or a homeless person—she treated everyone equally, and if she thought she was right, then look out! I am sure I channelled her voice at that moment. I started slowly and with more confidence than I'd had in weeks. "That is your opinion and I respect and value your medical opinion. But I am the baby's mother. I am the one who was given this child to carry and protect. I am not choosing to terminate this pregnancy and I will never choose that. This choice was mine and mine alone and this conversation is over. We are not discussing this option again." I was keeping this baby and if God took this one from me, then they would join my other children in heaven. There would be no more mention of options and if anything happened, I said, then I had confidence I could handle it.

Everything went quiet and when I looked at my husband and realized he was still looking down but now smiling. I was unwavering and I kept staring. Finally, she conceded and said that we should check the baby's heartbeat. That sound of the baby's heartbeat, that beautiful thumping, drowned out every sound and every doubt. It was the best sound in the whole world. The sound of a stadium full of applause couldn't match it. It was the best sound ever. *Don't worry, little one—I got you. We are going to be OK.*

Chapter 8
The Final Months—More Challenges

THE OB REMAINED POSITIVE THROUGHOUT OUR LAST FEW appointments and the memory of that conversation seemed to be a forgotten topic.

It was just over a month away from our due date when we met with our OB. At this point, you can almost let your guard down and let yourself believe. During this appointment, we were to pre-register at the hospital. We didn't have a choice of hospital. Because of our "high-risk" status, we had to go to the Royal Alex Hospital. We were excited about the pre-registration because it confirmed that we were close to meeting our baby. At the appointment, the doctor advised us that she wanted to delay our pre-registration. We were confused. "I think at this point we should be cautious and wait a few more weeks to register at the hospital. Also, because of your history, we will not be doing a final ultrasound."

I looked at her with disbelief and looked down at my obviously large pregnant stomach, which looked like a giant medicine ball at this point. I shifted as one of the kicks landed in my lower back and caused a jolt of pain in the area I would come to known as the sciatica.

With some trepidation, I asked exactly what we were being cautious about. "Well, given the complications you have experienced during this pregnancy . . ." *Complications*, aha, here was the forgotten topic rearing its head again.

"We should be open about the viability of the fetus." This is doctor-speak for *We don't think your baby will live. Excuse me? What do you mean? You said everything was fine and the heartbeat was strong and now you are bringing this up again. We thought we were going to pre-register today and it was going to be an exciting day and one of celebration. We just finished ten weeks of prenatal classes. We are at the point where we are finally excited about meeting our baby. We have the baby room set up and we bought baby shirts! And now we are talking about the viability of the fetus again????* I was stunned. I was shocked.

She continued, "We shouldn't expect this baby to weigh very much—it will be three pounds if we are lucky." What? I looked down at my extremely swollen belly, which looked like I could be carrying five babies. I was in complete shock.

"I think you should consider that this baby has undergone great adversity," she said.

"That is true," I said, "but I believe a higher power is on our side." Although doctors act like they have all the answers when you throw the higher power reference out, they really dislike it. "Doctor, I truly believe that." She sighed as she conceded that this conversation wasn't going anywhere. She briefly glanced at my husband, who was intensely staring at his shoes, and she knew she was not getting any support. "Let's just hope for the best. See you next week," she chimed, as she turned and headed out with the final word.

We are just going to have show her, I announced to my husband as I struggled to get off the hospital bed. *We will show her—this kid is going to stroll out and start telling jokes.* We both laughed.

One of the things they do not discuss in any great deal in any of the pregnancy books is the last two months of your pregnancy. For instance, they talk about the onset of labour. You will know when you start your labour, they say, because your mucous plug will dislodge. Like you even know what a mucous plug is—there is no picture of it in any of the books—just some vague description of a mucous gelatinous substance. I have a wild imagination and when I read that I immediately thought of the green blob from the *Ghostbusters* movie. Umm, nope. So, it has got to be obvious, right? As we look at each other in mock terror and optimism.

Contractions are the obvious onset of labour. Wrong again. Starting to get the idea that this isn't so textbook? You have been having Braxton Hicks contractions, which are fake contractions. I am not making this up. They feel real and, by that, I mean painful, and you go to the hospital thinking you are in labour. They can only discover they are Braxton Hicks by the evidence of your non-dilation. What they don't tell you is that they make you feel incredibly foolish. They will mock you and laugh and point. It will be middle school all over again. Trust me on this. Like everybody knows those aren't real—well, they *feel* real. They are extremely painful and sharp and take your breath away. You should time them, they advise. Well, if you are by yourself—good luck. That won't happen, as that jolt of pain and cramp hits you in your not-so-tiny belly and freezes you in your tracks as you try to survive until it subsides. Then you are panting and thinking, *Good God, that is going to happen again???* As these contractions are happening, you start to wonder when you go into the hospital. This was the biggest point of debate in the final weeks of pregnancy. Are these contractions real? Are the contractions just Braxton Hicks again? As we pondered the decision to go into the hospital or not, I announce I don't want the nurses to make fun of me again. I don't want to be cruelly mocked as I try to clumsily explain how *real* they felt and how much they *hurt*. It makes them laugh louder.

After we arrived home after our second Braxton Hicks incident, I declared to my husband, *we are not going to the hospital again until you can see the baby's head. I am not going through that again.* "And don't tell your mother!" I loudly declare as I hear him head for the phone. I don't want to hear that when *her* water broke, she not only mopped it up but cleaned all her floors before she drove herself to the hospital—only to have the doctor declare that she was already eight centimetres dilated when she arrived. Now this was her second child and, knowing my mother-in-law, there is not a part of that story that I don't believe. She has had five children, she is an amazing cook and baker, and her floors and house are in immaculate condition. She personally sands her hardwood floors and stains them every year. This is the ultimate housemaker and, yes, she would drive herself and sew herself back up. The last thing I needed was to hear the mocking disdain of her tone as she subtly pointed out that I was not her. No kidding.

My pastime during the last month of pregnancy was to pore over the books again and again. I was the equivalent of a beached whale and doing anything was completely exhausting. It was quite the spectacle when I left the house—as my poor husband would attempt to pull my body out of our little sedan. Even the little things became impossible. Like shaving your legs when you can't even see your legs. Like clipping your toenails because you don't want to go into labour splayed out for the world to see with long monster toenails and hairy bush-woman legs. So, your husband does it. It is humiliating.

And while I am being honest and real with you, wiping yourself 100 times per day when you dribble pulls muscles and resembles a bad Cirque Du Soleil move. So, you are *ginormous*, and your baby is pushed up practically into your throat, so your stomach is small and pushed so far down that the baby is residing on your bladder, which I am pretty sure resembles a deflated balloon at this point. So, you get this jabbing pain below the bulge, and you know you need to pee, so you wobble as quickly as you can to the washroom. It comes quickly and, since you are quickly losing control of those Kegel muscles, you pee yourself. Yes, ladies, you will pee yourself. It is humiliating—you will end up on the bathroom floor crying because of it and utterly embarrassed as you explain to your husband that he must clean up another dribble mess. But there is no way you are getting down on the floor to clean it and getting back up. Even if you weren't filled with shame and crying like a baby. I can tell you with confidence this tablespoon of pee will feel like a massive amount dribbling down your leg.

Last point: sleep or lack thereof. Sleeping is very hard in the last few months. You can't sleep lying down because you can't lie down horizontally if you ever expect to get up again without breaking your back. So, you prop yourself up in a bed or a recliner with pillows around you for some mild comfort.

Chapter 9

The Day We Finally Meet You!

I WAS LYING IN BED LIKE A BEACHED WHALE WHEN I SUDDENLY felt a stab of pain. Oh, no! I had to pee. Ugh. I tried to push myself up and roll over and fall off the bed. I wobbled to the washroom—panting like I was a running deer or black bear through the forest.

Whoosh. That was unmistakable!

Definitely! That was my water breaking. I pored over those pregnancy books and another thing they fail to mention is that, once your water breaks, it continues to leak. Yep, that's right. I realized this as I threw the tenth towel under me and scrambled for a pad. Then I meandered over to try and get dressed. I pulled on light pink overalls—the only things that fit me—with a T-shirt. I looked like a giant toddler. I hope that maternity clothes have changed. I had two options for maternity clothing: either look like a giant toddler or like I was wearing my grandmother's curtains. Then I waddled downstairs, still leaking constantly as I struggled to put my flip flops on. My feet were like swollen sausages at this point, and constantly felt like they were asleep. Funny, I didn't remember reading about that in my pregnancy books either.

My husband frantically came in and I said that my water had broken, and we were going to the hospital.

"Are you sure?" he asked, as he tripped on our labour bag at the front door. He was clearly starting to panic.

"Yes, I am."

At this point, a sense of calmness came over me and I felt oddly focused on what had to happen that day. I would get to meet my baby. As I struggled to sit in the front seat, my husband frantically ran around the car.

I looked at the labour bag and thought: *What a ridiculous thing.* In our prenatal class, they said you needed a labour bag, but I can tell you that, though this may be a great idea in theory, for us it became the joke about how many times the doctors and nurses could trip on it during the next twenty-four hours.

Why do you have a towel? my husband asked, suddenly noticing the towel I was sitting on.

Because my water broke, and I was still leaking.

What? my husband exclaimed; *the books didn't say that.*

Oh, really? I say sarcastically.

After we arrived at the hospital, we were escorted to a pre-birthing room. This is basically a ward with other beds where you can hang around and wait. I am not sure what I was expecting, but this wasn't it. A nurse came in and asked to examine me and I was propped in the uncomfortable familiar female position on my back. After a brief internal exam, she declared that I was two centimetres dilated and progressing nicely. As she left, she said that someone would be with me shortly.

Our hospital is a teaching hospital and there were many people coming in and out of the rooms. It was a flurry of activity and people, and you could feel ignored and invisible as they had many conversations among themselves. I always asked who they were and why they were there and, trust me, they didn't always announce themselves.

For instance, this one intern came in and, without a word, told me to open my legs. I asked him who he was and why he was there. He proceeded without saying anything, so I put my legs down and attempted to sit up. I said, "Who are you?" in a low voice that said, *I can bet you my day is going to be worse than yours, so answer me or scoot out of here*. He said he was there to break my water and started to push at my legs with this long metal instrument. "Get out," I said. "My water broke five hours ago."

"Are you sure?" he asked. "My notes say I have to break your water." He continued his task of attempting to skewer me with this silver stick.

"Get away from me—*now*," I said in a low, almost demonic, voice—*I heard it and I admit it*. Everything I had been through, and this little pipsqueak was not going anywhere near my baby, or I would skewer him. I got up and he checked my chart. "Wrong room," he said and ran out.

I was still rattled by my intern encounter when my contractions started. They came hard and fast. It was nothing like I could have imagined. Nothing like I had read. It was a piercing, excruciating pain in my back and stomach, like someone was trying to split me in two. Like a bad magic show act. I couldn't breathe it was agonizing. Time had no meaning.

Then it stopped. "Was that a contraction?" my husband asked. Truthfully, I am not a quiet woman, and I am known to use profanities, but one thing I am proud of is that I didn't curse or yell at my husband during labour. Still, at that moment, I came close.

"Holy bloody hell," I said. "That was a contraction and I hope they don't get worse." And just then another one hit! I was paralyzed in this incredible wave of pain, struggling for air.

"Remember your breathing," he said.

"Honestly, are you trying to test me? Are you kidding? I can't breathe—there will be no hoos and hees today. Get the nurse!!! Now!!"

Yup, that low, demonic voice came out again.

"Can you lie down?" the nurse asked, so she could hook me up to a baby monitor and a pain monitor. "Now, lying down is hard—remember—beached whale but in the threat of that intense wave of pain—how do you do that?" I headed toward the bed and, whoosh, another wave of pain—nobody touches me!

"Breathe," the nurse chided. I glared at her (and I know it was a murderous stare), and she backed off. The contraction subsided and I continued to get into bed, determined to do so before the next wave hit. The nurse said, "You can't be so dramatic, you are just early in your labour." Now, I know there are a lot of great nurses out there and I have had some great ones help me through some really hard times, but this was not one of them. She grabbed my arm so hard and tried to yank me. "Let go of me," I said—my demonic voice was useful at this point, and I was embracing it. Then another contraction hit, and she was irritated that it hindered her efforts to put on these monitors. It felt like every part of my body was vibrating with this pain and I didn't want anyone touching me when I was going through it.

She finally put the monitors on, and I heard the soothing sound of that heartbeat—*thump ker—thump ker—there you are, little one*. Oh, God, are you feeling this wave? —*It is intense. We got this, little one!* "This has got to be wrong," the nurse announced after one of my waves of pain. "Your contractions are a minute long and less than a minute apart."—*Yep, no kidding*. "And they are registering at the top of the pain metre for intensity." *Again—I know!!!*

"I am sorry, do you want anything for pain?" Another wave hit and I was withdrawing into myself to survive these waves.

"Is that OK?" she asked.

"What? I said.

"I just gave you morphine—ten millilitres."

"Really? When?"

"Just a minute ago."

"Huh? No effect. Zero effect."

When you are in labour, you have no sense of time or anything else going on around you. At least that was my experience. I would breathe outward with a vibrating hum while the contractions happened and, after, I would try to catch my breath and to breathe normally and calmly. This is all very relative to the state you are in, by the way.

At one point—over six hours into it—my favourite nurse mentioned my humming noise was upsetting my husband and said I should stop it. I looked at my husband and he looked at me with this sense of panic on his face and declared quickly, "I didn't say that." *I know we have been through a lot and there is no way this is upsetting him and, quite frankly, I don't care at that point in time.* Out came my demonic voice again and I said, "Get out!" I was focused solely on the sound of the heartbeat as I got through another five hours of this cycle (so I was told afterward—I had no sense of time, remember?).

It came time to push and at some point, they put an epidural in me which I have no recollection of. Also, my husband and my doctor went to McDonald's for a bite to eat which I have no recollection of, and he foolishly confessed this to me afterwards. I was in the awkward position of the legs raised when the doctor announced it was time to push and, with the next contraction, I did—for another ten times. The head was stuck, the doctor said. "Let's try forceps," he said, but they didn't work. "Let's try . . . mutter, mutter, mutter." The muttering resulted in my pelvic bone breaking, so I was glad to have missed that. While this hustle was going on—I was focusing on the baby's heartbeat—and then it stopped!

I sat up and was on high alert! I was fully conscious and aware and full of panic. The room was in complete silence, and everyone realized what had happened. In an instant—and I really mean in a split second—everyone broke into action. I was rushed out of this room and down the hall, with a lot of yelling and chattering. I was back to my chant of *Please be OK, little one—hang in there. Please, we got this.* Then we were in the operating room and, since I already have an epidural in, they started the C-section. Suddenly, there was an intense burning pain on my stomach—Oh, God, I can feel them slicing me open. "I can feel that" I said. They looked at each other and continued, convinced I couldn't. They were hyper-focused on the task at hand. I felt them opening my stomach and I told them I could feel them pulling at the incision. They suddenly realized that I *could* feel it and called for the anesthesiologist to put me out. "Get the husband out of here," they said, and he was rushed out and they put me under. *I can't hear the heartbeat—please let it be OK*, I thought, as I drifted away.

When I woke up, my first thought was: *My baby*. I was only vaguely aware of my head at this point and had no conscious thought of where I was or where my body was. "Your son is fine, a voice said, as she put a baby next to my face and he looked at me with the biggest, bluest eyes I had ever seen. "Hello, little one—we made it. You OK? Those eyes! I am so happy that you have my nose!! I am so happy to meet you." Then I slipped into unconsciousness again.

When I awoke some six hours later, I thought: *Did I dream that? Where is my baby? Did I have a baby? What happened? Was it a dream?* "My baby?" I managed to say with a croaked voice. "Take it easy," the nurse said—*Nope, not until I see my baby.*

"Please, I have to know."

"He is fine. He is a perfectly healthy ten-pound baby boy."

What?? "Please, I need to see him." This is something I think only a mom could truly understand. You *need* to see your baby. You cannot take anyone's word for it—you want to be able to see them to know that they are OK. We waited ten months to see them, and nothing can ease the anxiety until we do. I am not sure if all new moms feel this way or just the ones that experience such worry or complications during the pregnancy. But *I needed to see him.*

When they brought him to me, I could only stare at him. I looked up at my husband and smiled.

"We did it. Is he really OK?"

"Yes," he said.

"He is really ours?"

"Yes," he said.

"He is perfect, isn't he?"

"Absolutely." He grinned. "Honey, you should know something."

"Nope, at this moment I just want to stare at him." He was perfect—absolutely 100 percent perfect. At that moment, I felt like I had climbed Everest, and it was the greatest feeling in the world.

Chapter 10
The Hours After Birth

I READ A LOT OF BABY BOOKS AND VERY FEW OF THEM COVERED what happens after you give birth. No one really tells you the details of it. It all comes as quite a shock and people look at you like you have been downloaded this information as a woman. Like at some point you have been given all this information that you just should automatically know. *Didn't your mother tell you?* is the incredulous question. *Are you kidding me?*

My mother was an open woman and, unlike 95 percent of the mothers during the time of my upbringing, she talked openly about boys and kissing and even sex, to a point. She was a wonderfully funny and open woman, and I am grateful to her for so many things. However, a big caveat here, women who grew up in the fifties and sixties did not speak of certain things. A woman didn't speak of your period—it was an unspoken rule. Like hiding when you were on your period and not discussing "your time" or "Aunt Flo visiting." I didn't have the talk about my period, and I honestly thought I was dying when I got it, but that is another story.

If no one talked about what happens after birth and it isn't covered in detail in pregnancy books, how are you supposed to find out? It is truly like a secret club. Of course, woman who have experienced childbirth know what happens afterwards but nope—we don't talk about it. So, I am talking about it because I am carrying on the tradition of being a rule breaker. Thanks Mom.

To review, I had a C-section after trying to deliver vaginally. One fact is that the nurses will classify you as *either* a natural birth or a C-section birth—no chance of crossover, which I didn't know until I tried to go to the washroom. But let me back up, to the point of trying to get up out of bed. I immediately was aware of the searing pain across my abdomen. Oh, yeah, *that*! They cut a gash across your stomach in this procedure—in my case, two. You are left with a giant, flabby stomach that still looks like you are five months pregnant. It was a shock for me because I recall women on TV with their skinny jeans on after giving birth.

So, after a few hours, they want to get you up and walking. Going to the washroom is the first goal. So, they announce it to you like you are a six-year-old—*We are going to get up and go to the washroom, OK?* They ask you to swing your legs off the bed. *There is no swinging.* With your stomach feeling like a ton of bricks combined with searing pain across your abdomen, there is no swinging. You are moving slowly and methodically. Or at least I was.

I attempted to sit up on the edge of the bed and was completely exhausted. Then the nurse announced, "OK, let's stand up! Now, sure, standing up is something we have all done, but I hadn't seen my legs or feet in months, and I am not completely sure I had full feeling or control of them at this point. But because she had the tone of my condescending second-grade teacher, I attempted to stand. I had very little strength at this point, and I was very weak. So, standing was not super easy and I was grasping at everything. Also, around this point, I was starting to feel extremely nauseous, so I was breathing in and out, trying not to be nauseous and using every bit of your awareness and strength to stand.

OK, we are standing!! I feel it is upright, but I know I am slouched as I can only see the floor. Well, upright is upright and I am taking the win. "OK, now let's walk slowly," the nurse announced because, at this point, someone has obviously started to run down the hall. Your body is going to feel extremely weird. Remember, the last recollection you had was the beached whale who waddled. Now you have a giant, flabby thing that is your stomach, and your body is extremely swollen and still doesn't quite feel like it is yours.

We started the slow meander toward the washroom. I felt this searing pain in my stomach, and it felt like flames were shooting out of me. I attempted to put my hand on my stomach with my free hand. "You are doing great," the nurse announced. And I looked at her like I knew she was lying. Shuffle, shuffle, you move, because you aren't lifting your feet to walk so much as dragging and shuffling them, completely unsure if they can even support you.

Then you finally make it to the washroom, and they want you to sit down. You are completely aware of the searing fire ring on your stomach and start to doubt your abdominal muscles. Oh, OK, the nursing is pushing you down. Sweet mother of #*#, that is excruciating, and you feel like passing out. The wave of nausea resembles the worst drinking night of your life, and the room starts to spin. You can't tell which way is up.

"OK, now let's pee," the nurse announced. *Honestly, can you make me feel more like a two-year-old or a puppy?* Then the searing pain of fire that followed was indescribable. "You are a C-section," the nurse said, because she recognized this was uncomfortable. Then she suddenly remembered that I'd had an episiotomy. "It is just a few stitches, dear." *What? Oh, God.* As I am struggling to wipe myself, my arms are too short, and I can't reach it. And you suddenly notice there is blood. *What is that?* "Oh, yeah," the nurse said. "That is normal." *What?* No one has mentioned this. And there is this weird strap-held pad that is like a small canoe. Another thing they don't tell you—you bleed afterward, like a heavy period, and it can last six weeks or more—a fun fact that I didn't read about in those baby books. Wait, maybe they said spotting—highly understated, once again.

Another piece of information that no one tells you is that you swell afterward. Let me be perfectly clear about this: *every* part of your body swells—your hands, your legs, your feet, your toes. *Everything.* And not just a little bit. We are talking the Michelin Man type of swelling. Not sure why, but you swell a lot, and you feel like your feet are asleep. For me, this swelling lasted for almost a week, but it really didn't go away for about three weeks.

Chapter 11
Grieving

AFTER MY FIRST MISCARRIAGE, I WAS DEVASTATED, AND nothing could have prepared me for the pain and emotions. I never wanted to go through that again. Sadly, it wasn't the only miscarriage that we would experience, and little did I know the path that was ahead of us. We had a long and painful road of miscarriages before I had my son and a few more before I had my daughter. Honestly, I am glad I didn't know because I wouldn't have had the strength to face it. If I had known that path, I may not have chosen it.

I found strength in my darkest moments and the strongest of all people are the moms who never get to hold their babies. We suffer losses in silence every day and never, ever forget the children we never got to meet. The Mother's Days, the Father's Days, the Christmases, and the birthdays they never get to have. Their first days of school. All those little life moments that remind you. Every time you see a mom with their baby, you are reminded that you didn't get to hold your baby and it hurts. You don't ever get over it. Time doesn't help. You remember them—even if it was only a few weeks or months into the pregnancy. They were your baby and you wanted them, and you loved them. And you always will. And you can never talk about them with other moms, and you can never bring them up with your family. You just remember them in silence and by yourself and you never ever forget them. It has been thirty years since I lost Matthew and I have never forgotten him. My eyes well up with tears as I write this as I remember that loss. It does matter and it wasn't just a peanut—he was my baby and I miss him. I couldn't protect him, and I couldn't save him and that hurts and cuts deeper that anyone can possibly imagine.

The plain truth is that I remember every one of my losses. I remember how many children I have lost along the way. I have named them all—I have mourned every one of them. I miss each one of them. It didn't get easier with each loss—it got harder. It was harder and harder each time to try again to think that it could be different—to dare to hope. I cried for every one of them and on every Mother's Day and every Christmas. I remember the children I will never hold and whose smiling faces I will never get to see and whose tears I will never get to wipe. I remember every one of my children and I cry for each one of them, even decades after I had to say goodbye. *I remember all of you and I look forward to the day when I can meet all of you again. What a party that will be! What a day that will be.*

That is the truth and I pray that you don't know what I am talking about—that you never do, and if you do know then I am sorry and I mourn with you for the child you can never hold and never meet. For the loss you must pretend you don't feel and can never show to the world. I hug each one of you as you cry in private for the children lost—for all the hopes and dreams for those children that were taken too soon, without warning or condolence.

Whether you have been pregnant for a day, a week, or five months, you lost your baby. Never mind about science or any other description. This was *your baby*. From that first day of finding out, you became a mom and a dad, and your every thought was about the baby. When that baby's life ended prematurely, it was devasting. I like the word *prematurely* better than "loss" and "miscarriage," which feel like you are referring to something insignificant, like your keys. You lose your keys. You don't lose your baby. The baby's life ends. Your baby's life.

It is heartbreaking and it feels like a piece of your heart has been pulled from your chest. And it isn't like a normal death—there isn't a funeral or a cast of supporting family surrounding you and helping you with your loss. If you are lucky, your partner is beside you—mourning your loss. If he isn't by your side—believe that he is mourning this loss, too, in his own way. It isn't a public mourning; it is very much private. Family and friends will dismiss and minimize it. *It was only the size of a peanut. Just start over. It is fun making the babies, isn't it? It wasn't like it was alive, it was just a fetus.* That your friends and family say these insensitive things isn't their fault. They don't understand. No one can hope to ever understand it unless they have been through it. And in our mothers' generation, you didn't discuss miscarriages. You had to deal with them alone and move forward. This makes them even more painful and hard to deal with.

The one thing that stuck with me was that this baby wasn't real for everyone. It was so very real for us, and the loss was deeply felt. I had to make it real, so we had something to grieve. We named all our babies, and I also wrote them each a letter. I know many mothers have done this and found comfort. I wrote how I was so excited when we found out about them. That, even though we thought that we would never be able to sleep in, it was OK—we would have such fun together. Playing and sledding. I wrote down all my thoughts and dreams for them. Then after I had said everything I needed to, I told them that we would meet again one day. That they would always be with me. And I promised never to forget them. I said they were my child—my son or my daughter—and I would always love them, even though we couldn't be together now. I buried these letters, but I can remember every word. (I have included a few letters in the last chapter). I didn't need a physical reminder. I would never forget them.

We had private funerals for each of them, burying a sleeper or toy we had picked out in their box along with their special letter. Saying a few words and planting a tree or flower over the spot.

We chose to remember them in little ways. The first Christmas after my first loss, my husband gave me a gift of a porcelain doll named Matthew. He was wearing the cutest sailor suit and he had the cutest face and little smile. Every time I look at it, I think of him, and that brings me comfort in his memory. Every Christmas after that, he gave me a gift for the one we had lost, porcelain dolls or stuffed animals—they became our secret gift at Christmas. I felt like he was remembering our babies and that made me happy. No one understood my collection of porcelain dolls and stuffed animals and that is OK. *This remembrance is for you.* Plant a tree, plant a flower, draw a picture—however you need to express and remember that baby. No judgement. No pressure. If it takes a week, a month, or a year for you to mourn them, it is not wrong. It is your loss and your grief. It is real and it is yours.

There are many levels of pain during these experiences. The obvious one is the grief of the loss of the baby you can never hold or meet. The other part is the loneliness and frustration over the lack of answers and support. It isn't something anyone can talk about. The medical community offers little information of the experience; they are just treating a condition. So goes their medical training, and I have the greatest respect for these professionals and the work they do. When I expressed concern to my doctor whenever I got pregnant again, the doctor's response was whether to continue the pregnancy or not. They recommended talking to a psychologist, but I did not find it helpful. I relieved these painful experiences to a stranger who had never experienced it and in the end, it offered me no comfort or answers.

These are only my experiences of dealing with grief over my babies. There is no wrong way to grieve, and it isn't quick and simple. There are moments, years afterward, that will bring this pain and grief back to the surface. It is a hole in your heart that will always be there. People will say time heals everything, and that will be a lie. I can tell you it has been almost thirty years since my first loss, and I still vividly remember and feel that loss. As I am writing this, I am blinking back tears for the babies I will meet someday in heaven.

I will end this chapter on a positive note. I have since learned that there are baby-loss support groups and I encourage you to reach out to them. It is a comfort knowing someone has gone through this, too, and they won't offer any judgement about your loss. Whether your loss is an early miscarriage or a stillborn, it is still a great loss. I have found talking with mothers who have experienced such losses offers an understanding and compassion that you will seldom find anywhere else.

Chapter 12
The Dads

I KNOW THAT WOMEN CARRY THE BABIES, BUT ALONGSIDE them and often forgotten are the dads. They were barely even mentioned in my pregnancy books.

I read somewhere that a man becomes a father once he meets his baby. I would like to amend this adage. I believe that men become dads at that moment of the positive pregnancy test. Because their every thought is about the baby and what is best for them. And their wife also becomes something more in that moment. She becomes the mother of your child, and they immediately feel more protective of her. Your perspective on, thoughts of, and feelings toward her are forever changed. In that instant, that baby is yours—real in your heart and in your mind.

My husband would vehemently declare that he didn't think about the pregnancy every moment of every day. A fact that made me angry and resentful towards him. Since then, I have come to realize that this is simply not true. In fact, he did constantly think about the pregnancy and worry just as much as I did. That is right, men—I am calling you out. You become invested in that baby from the moment of the positive pregnancy test, too. If pregnancy loss is not talked about or acknowledged with women, it is talked about even less among men. I must reiterate at this point that this is simply *my* experience, and bravo if you have had a more positive experience.

As much as women are expected to know about all things baby because it is our bodies, there are also high expectations for men. The doctors and specialists look to them for answers and insight. They are asked to make impossible choices and informed of situations and left to deal with the aftermath. They are given no tools and no support and no information. They have a front-row seat to the carnage, and they are expected to be strong and hopeful and offer the right words of encouragement or defence. It is quite an impossible predicament.

We have thankfully made progress from my parents' generation (Boomers), when the fathers were not invited to the OB appointments or into the birthing room (so how were they expected to know anything about pregnancy or birth?). They typically didn't offer any advice or have any conversations with their sons. They simply didn't talk about women's issues, such as carrying children and birthing. The result was a generation of men who had no support system or information for dealing with the impossible task of navigating pregnancy challenges and complications.

Imagine for a second how hard it was for these Gen-X men to ask questions about a miscarriage or discuss how hurt they felt afterward. It was met with silence or, worse, laughter and insults. The "walk it off, son" and the "man up" and the "just deal with it" approaches are lacking and cruel.

After a few miscarriages, my husband went to speak with a therapist as he was feeling a mixture of things about the experiences and didn't feel like he could talk to anyone. He was angry with me for putting him through the miscarriages and understandably felt like he couldn't discuss his feelings with me. He also felt completely helpless to help me or the baby we had lost and angry, with nowhere to put that anger.

As hard as it was for me to endure the family conversations and people's dismissive and judgemental glares it was even harder for him. Even I didn't recognize the extra strain on him and helplessness he felt. He had a front-row seat to the experience and watched helplessly as I miscarried plus dealt with my onslaught of emotions and anger. I didn't realize that he felt attached to and protective of the baby, too, and couldn't do anything to prevent the miscarriage. He had the added strain of watching the person he loved the most go through pain and felt he couldn't even offer simple comfort or take away any of the pain. I had no idea how hard it was for him, and I didn't even try to see his perspective at the time. Ironically, he felt as alone as I did in his grief and loss.

He confessed to me later that it was hard to watch me go through everything (the miscarriages and the complications) and to not know what to do or say. He said he knew he couldn't do or say anything that was going to help, and it was ripping him apart inside. He never told me at the time. I wish he had, but I understand why he didn't.

At the fertility appointments, he confessed that he hated that he felt dismissed and diminished. I was shocked when he revealed this to me as I remember being angry at how little attention was on him. But I never thought about how that made him feel. He said that he felt reduced to a sperm donor. In appointments, they deferred to him only when things went sideways, and they expected him to make decisions with little or no information. He felt it was an unfair and impossible situation, plus he knew it was adding to how upset I was.

After miscarriages, no one asked him if he wanted to try again, and I never even considered him in the decision. He never got to process his grief and any questions were only about how I was doing. He felt invisible. He felt selfish and insensitive for even thinking that he should be given consideration. There was no support system for him, and he was caught in the middle of defending me and keeping the peace with his family. I never considered how hard it was for him at the time. If I wasn't shown how to grieve as woman over the loss of my child, he certainly wasn't given any skills or even permission to grieve. I am grateful that we had these conversations, and he was able to begin his healing journey.

I would be remiss if I didn't mention the strain on the relationship and marriage. A miscarriage is a hard event to recover from physically and emotionally. There are many complicated layers to the experience, and it really does affect your relationship. Multiple miscarriages are an exponential strain, and they certainly took their toil on us.

This part was a surprise revelation for me. There is some resentment toward the mom from the husband. They want someone to blame, and we are the ones carrying the baby. I don't say this lightly, but those feelings are real. But how could we not know what was happening with our bodies? How could we prevent it? If this is a mystery to a woman, then it's an inexplicable conundrum to a man. This is even more compounded when you think of their mothers and family stories. Most of their mothers have stories of easy childbirth and popping out multiple children. I mean, who hasn't heard the ploughing-the-field story of a grandmother who gave birth and continued working? Large families with ten or more children were common for our grandmothers. Their stories are strong developmental memories for men. Their mothers are their only example of motherhood in all areas of their life. The mothers were strong pillars of the family and none of their difficulties were ever discussed. Understandably, this had a strong impact on their sons' impression of motherhood and the experience of miscarriage is a direct shock to that foundation.

Of course, our mothers and grandmothers lost children, too, but it was never talked about. I mean, it was easy—or so it seemed to be—for so many people to get pregnant and have babies. If women can't wrap their heads around miscarriages then men have less of a chance to. Resentment and questions are all part of their grieving process. But husbands can't admit it because that would be insensitive and mean after what the mom went through. But it is the truth.

When I gave birth to my son, my husband was kicked out the operating room. He was told that he could lose both of us and to choose. An impossible choice. In my father's generation, I can almost understand the black-and-white answer of "save the mother—she can always have more children." Having children was a function of a woman and what she was born to do. A simple choice for them but I wonder how many of them would admit it wasn't that simple. Different generation and different experiences. But in that moment when my husband was asked to choose, he simply said the baby. *Save the baby.* Of course, he said that. We had spent months wishing and praying this baby was OK. He was angry that he had to make that choice. He was angry that he came close to losing his wife and our baby. He was angry that he had been robbed of the experience that our friends talked about and that he had seen on TV and in the movies. This is not what he thought this day would look like. This was supposed to be a joyous occasion and once again he felt completely robbed.

It was unfair. It is OK to be angry about that—it is natural, even if no one tells you that. *I* will tell you that. You are going through the experience, and you get to feel what you feel, and you shouldn't be judged or questioned. The dads always joke that the birth was a tough for them and say they did a great job and congratulate each other. I used to joke how silly that was, but I understand their perspective better now. The dads aren't just spectators, supporting cast members, or sperm donors.

My husband was completely aware of everything going on and heard the conversations that I missed in my pain-riddled state. He felt the anxiety and panic, too, but throughout it all felt like an invisible spectator completely left out and barely considered.

I applaud all the dads out there for everything they go through supporting the moms and offer a personal apology to my husband—twenty years too late—for everything he went through

Chapter 13
Closing Thoughts

IT IS MY SINCERE HOPE THAT YOU FOUND SOME ANSWERS AND comfort from my story. This book has been over twenty years in the making. These types of experiences were rarely discussed or talked about twenty years ago. When I would offer an empathic ear to women who'd experienced losses, they would encourage me to write a book so all women would have access to this information.

I thank those women for their support and encouragement. In this book, I have truly re-opened the most painful and personal experiences of my life and have relived them in detail with the sincere hope that it offers some comfort and empathy. It is truly an exclusive club of women who experience the loss of a baby, and we are a strong, silent group. I hope that this book breaks that silence, and that miscarriage becomes a mainstream topic for mothers and fathers alike.

My heart goes out to all mothers and fathers who have gone through the pain and loss of an empty crib and who never got to hold those children who reside in heaven.

Chapter 14

Letters To My Unborn Children

Dear Matthew:

You were only in our life a short time, but I wanted you to know how much you changed us.

We used to think about sleeping in on the weekends and lazing in bed all day watching TV. When we first found out we were pregnant, we thought about that at first. How silly that seems now.

Our second thought and every thought after that was about you. How much we were excited about how our life would change and how every day would be so fun. We would go for walks in the park and to the playground when you got older. We would go swimming and teach you how to swim. We love the water and I know you would have too. We talked about picnics and camping and imagined just lying-in bed with you, watching you sleep.

We wondered what you looked like. If you had my nose instead of your father's hook. If you had my eyes or my mom's. If you would be silly or if you would be serious. We wondered if you would be a beautiful baby girl, or a handsome little boy and your father smiled at the thought of both. If you would love the zoo or watching baseball. Every day we thought of you. I thought of you with my every waking thought and my last thought at night.

Too soon we had to say goodbye. I prayed and wished with all my heart and soul that you could have stayed with us. It already felt like you were a part of our life and you filled us with such joy and excitement. Every moment of every day I miss you. You are still my first thought every morning and my last thought every night. Little one, I hope to meet you one day in heaven so we can do all the things we dreamt of. We miss you and we will love you always. Just know we really wanted you with every breath and thought. We were a family for a very short time, and I want to thank you for that. A part of my heart went to heaven with you that day you left. You will never be forgotten.

All my love, your mom—if only for a short time.

Dear Mark and David,

Today we had to say goodbye to you and way too soon. They told us that you were twins after. I want you to know that I prayed and wished, and I did everything right. I don't know what happened. I did everything the doctor asked. But I don't want you to worry about that. I know you are safe and happy now in heaven.

I wanted you to know that we were so excited to meet you and how great it would have been to have twin boys. We pictured how cute you both would have looked, one with big blue eyes and blonde hair and maybe the other with brown eyes and brown hair. Both with distinct personalities and looks.

I know you liked to dance in my tummy when I played the radio loud and danced around. I know you would have had my love of music. I would have loved that. I would have encouraged you to take music lessons and play an instrument. Maybe the piano and maybe we could have learned together.

We thought of you every day and there wasn't a moment that went by when we weren't talking about how much fun we would have together. Sledding in the park and swimming lessons on Saturday. How we would dress you up in a cute outfit for Halloween and take lots of pictures that would be totally embarrassing. You would have laughed at us and forgiven us because secretly you would have thought it was funny, too.

I miss you both so much. You were a part of our lives for seventeen weeks and I enjoyed every second of it. We had even picked out a few sleepers to take you home from the hospital in. You both will always be in our hearts and thoughts. You will always be our sons and I promise to think of you every Christmas and everyday—even fifty years from now. You will always be in our hearts—please know that.

I love you with every piece of my heart, which is why you can take a piece with you for safekeeping.

Till we meet again—your mom on earth.

All my love

Charlene Robertson

Thank you to my Angel Team and for all their divine inspiration and help writing this book. I know the strength to write these stories was a gift from you. May I always be in service of the divine white light.

With so much gratitude and love.